PLAN YOUR DIET
LIKE AN EXPERT

BY

AKANKSHA SHARMA

THE FITNESS KEY SERIES

(BOOK-1)

Copyright Statement

In the loving memory of my Naani (Late Smt. Prem Lata Sharma), may her memory forever be a comfort and blessing.

Acknowledgement

I dedicate this book to my daughter (Dakshayini Gupta) and my husband (Abhishek Gupta).

Any accomplishment requires the effort of many people and this work is no different. I am indeed blessed with a lot of wonderful people in my life. Without them, I could not have written my dream book.

I would like to express my gratitude to all of them for their support and love. There are no words to express my gratitude to my father (Mr. Dinesh Sharma), my mother (Mrs. Nisha Sharma), and my sister (Miss Esha Sharma) for their unconditional love, support and motivation.

I would also like to express my gratitude towards my father-in-law (Mr. Raj Kumar Gupta) and mother-in-law (Mrs. Anju Gupta) who have always encouraged me to move ahead in life. I feel grateful to my aunt (Mrs. Pooja Goel) for being my support system throughout this journey.

I feel grateful to my husband (Abhishek Gupta) for his faith and foresight to see the potential in me always. I will also like to thank him for his patience and moral support; whenever I asked him for support, he never turned me down. He has always stood behind me in all of my endeavors.

I am also thankful to all other family members and friends who have always been a source of inspiration to me. I wish to express my gratitude to those who may have contributed to this work, even though anonymously.

I also want to express my gratitude to my editor, Olorunlowu Darasimi for editing this book. I really appreciate everyone, thank you so much.

Preface

With the increase in health issues due to environmental problems, sedentary lifestyle and poor eating habits, fitness has become an unavoidable need in everyone's life. I myself have experienced fatty liver issues, being overweight in the past, and I know how bad it feels to deal with them. Everybody has his/her journey, and mine is from fat to fab within one year of delivering a baby.

There are many people on my social handle who used to text me on how they can reduce their weight or maintain a healthy weight, and thereby my family and friends have encouraged me to write a book on my weight loss journey. And there on, I decided I should not only write a book on weight loss but the process it takes to a holistic fitness of a body.

With this book, I aim to make my readers so much capable that they can not only take care of themselves but also of their families. This book is for everyone who wants to see themselves and their family members fit and healthy. This book is also for those who are juggling with their confidence just because of overweight and underweight issues.

Being a nutritionist, I promise by the time you finish this book, you will be able to see yourself; how easy it is to lose or gain weight by yourself without spending money on expensive supplements or dieticians.

There are so many books on healthy eating, the importance of losing weight, balanced diets, readymade diets or specialized diets, but I have hardly seen any book that tells you the process of how you can plan your diet.

As it is wisely said that *"Give a man a fish and you feed him for a day, teach a man to fish and you feed him for a lifetime"*, with the help of this book, you will not only learn about the foods and approaches that can help you to lose weight; instead, this book aims at making you plan your diet like an expert.

With a baby of 1 year old, it was a challenge for me to write about my fitness journey. But I believe that motherhood gives wings to fly and you feel you are stronger than ever. I am thankful to my husband for his untimely support and making this happen. It wouldn't have been possible without his help. I am grateful to my baby girl also, Dakshayini who has always been my strength.

This book does not only aim at making you an expert in diet planning, but also make you aware of how the well nutritious balanced diet is essential for your health. A chapter has been incorporated in this book which deals with myths regarding weight loss and how you can you make your diet enjoyable by following some simple food hacks.

This book is my attempt to present the complex and vast subject called *"Diet planning"* in an easy-to-understand and enjoyable way so that anyone from any background can grasp the knowledge without any difficulties.

Almost all best-selling books on this topic are written based on some specific particular diets. Over the last few months, interactions with many of my clients helped me to realize the necessity to write a book solely based on diet planning. I think this book will serve the purpose.

The language used in this book is so simple that anyone from any background can understand it without any difficulties. Solely focused on Diet planning with many practical examples, this book will surely solve the purpose for those who are looking to learn the subject with minimum effort.

So, ask yourself:

- Are you looking for an easy-to-implement weight loss diet?
- Do you want to look smart, fit, confident and healthy in parties?
- Do you want to keep yourself and your family free from diseases and overweight issues?
- Does that postpartum weight gain haunt you?
- Do you want to come back to shape after delivering a baby?
- Don't have time for exercise but still want to lose weight fast?

If your answer to any of the questions above is "YES," then just go ahead. This book won't disappoint you.

Introduction

This book is a step by step guide to make you self-sufficient in planning your diet. It also includes a list of super foods, amazing food hacks, cheat meal ideas, and sample diet plans. This book is for everyone who wants to get back in shape quickly. If you are holding this book in your hands or you are reading on your kindle, that means you want to get rid of that extra fat, or you want to build muscles, or you want to maintain your current body shape.

I want to congratulate you as you have chosen the book that has been perfectly planned to help you achieve the desired body shape. This Book-1 of the Fitness Key Series is aimed at improving your health through planning a perfect diet by an excellent coach that is none other than you.

Plan Your Diet Like an Expert is book one of ***The Fitness Key Series*** which will help you to understand your body and metabolism. This book is designed to help you make your diet plan in five simple steps.

Various studies found that 39% of the global adult populations were classified as overweight or obese in 2014. The prevalence of overweight and obesity in

India is increasing faster than the world average. According to a study by the World Health Organization, it was found that 22% of women suffer from postpartum depression in India. Around 74% of urban Indians are overweight, and according to a survey conducted by Fitho; a leading wellness services organization, it was found that people are becoming aware of losing weight. Still, only 5 out of 10 are taking actions to get back into shape.

The book is for those who are ready to take action and believe in doing rather than finding excuses. This book will help you deal with problems of obesity, weight loss, weight management, and stuck pregnancy weight. It will bust all your myths related to weight loss, making it easier for you to understand how a perfectly planned diet can change your life, making you more confident about your appearance and thus giving you the more new avenues of success.

This book will guide you about the ways you can effectively monitor your calorie intake and help you to plan your diet according to it. This book deals with step by step process of diet planning, including some fantastic food hacks, methods to plan your cheat meal, the list of super foods and sample diet plans. Thus, this book is designed in a way so that you can plan your diet just like an expert.

"Give a man a fish, and you feed him for a day; teach a man to fish, and you feed him for a lifetime."

Table of Contents

PART I-Getting the Mindset Right

Chapter One – Myths Related to Weight Loss to be Busted

"A very pleasant surprise was the items I thought were naughty, but those that I enjoyed immensely like strong coffee, dark chocolate, nuts, high-fat yoghurt, wine and cheese, are likely to be healthy for me and my microbes"— **Tim Spector.**

People often tell you to do exercises to lose weight; to hit the gym as soon as possible, or to wake up early and go for running with your neighbor who runs a marathon. So here is an eye-opener; you don't need to do any of these against your will to get your dream body. Some myths need to be busted right away to make your mindset ready for this journey.

Diet means starving

I remember meeting a friend at a housewarming party where I noticed that he didn't have his dinner so I asked him;"is everything alright?" He told me that he is dieting and he planned to lose weight in a short time. I asked him about his purpose of doing that on which he told me that he wants to look smart on his wedding day which is just two months away.

On learning that I am a nutritionist, he discussed his plan with me to confirm whether he was on the right path or not. I asked him in detail about the diet schedule he was following and he told me he used to have a glass of milk in the morning, a bowl of boiled dal for lunch and a plate full of salad as dinner. I was shocked to hear that as he was just starving himself; denying himself the joy of the moment.

Moreover, this can cause a long-lasting irreparable damage to his body as eventually, he will be going short of essential nutrients and minerals in his body. He will surely lose weight very fast, but he was moving towards a life with low energy and that which is vulnerable to diseases.

I told him that as soon as he starts eating, he will gain back the fat more rapidly and distortedly. I counseled him thoroughly and prepared a personalized month diet plan that was varied and made to keep in mind his food choices. Now, he was eating more than before but according to his body's nutritional requirements. The results were unbelievable for him as within a week; he lost 2kgs without feeling low on energy and without starving himself at all. So, this is the common myth most of us have in our mind; that diet means eating less and starving to shed weight.

Diet means planning your meals according to your body's nutritional requirements, rather than eating less. Basically, it's a "eat more, loose more" approach. A proper diet plan includes 5-6 meals per day with a gap of 2-3hrs between each meal, and eating in small amounts frequently rather than eating in one go.

When I started planning my diet, I was eating much better foods the whole day and with a wide variety. So while planning a diet, I always remember that macronutrients (proteins, fats and carbs) are essential for the body. There is no generalized diet plan that suits everyone as many books suggest; every diet plan should be made according to the body of each person.

Proper knowledge or expert guidance is vital for diet planning, which you will be gaining yourself as you finished this book.

Weight loss becomes difficult with increasing age

A Choreographer and well-known dancer, Ganesh Acharya has lost 85kg in just 1.5 years at the age of

48, and has been an inspiration to all who believe the myth that weight loss is not possible at such age. If we see around ourselves, we'll indeed find someone we know who has also transformed his/her body after the age of 40 or 50.

My mother used to complain about her knee pain. She visited several doctors and they used to advise her to reduce at least 10kgs which seems to be impossible for her. But I made sure that she achieved this target of losing the extra kgs; I introduced some minor changes to her diet and her lifestyle. Within three months, she was able to reduce 10kgs, and she noticed that her knee pain began to reduce as she started feeling much better.

You may experience many lifestyle changes as you age, such as Retirement; it may reduce the amount of physical activities. After working throughout life, you may see retirement as an extended vacation. The relaxed schedule can make you indulge in unhealthy foods without the daily exercise.

I have seen people live a healthy, disease-free life rather than an overweight body with a pile of diseases. Effectively planning your diet may not only help you to lose weight at any age, but it also ensures that you remain less vulnerable to age-related diseases.

Pregnancy weight is difficult to reduce

After delivering my baby, my mother-in-law made sure that I was served gond laddoos and sheera as she believes that they will help in overcoming fatigue, weakness and also help in milk production. As far as these laddoos and post-pregnancy meals are concerned, they contain a lot of refined sugar which is bad for the health and a significant reason why you put on weight.

I did some minor changes to my meals by replacing sugar with jaggery; so instead of having sugary sheera, I tried jaggery and dry fruits energy bars, and I always made sure that my meals were cooked in desi ghee as I knew undoubtedly that ghee do miracles with weight loss.

According to the studies, it is found that most women lose about 13 pounds (5.9 kilograms) during childbirth, including the weight of the baby, placenta and amniotic fluid. During the first week after delivery, you'll lose additional weight as you shed retained fluids — but the fat stored during pregnancy won't disappear on its own, and these laddoos are very high in sugar content.

Focus more on eating fruits and vegetables rather than junk food as you get natural sugars from fruits. If you have a sweet tooth, keep some cubes of jaggery in your kitchen instead of ice creams, sweets and those flavored sugar syrups, as jaggery has more antioxidants and more health benefits.

Try to have 4-5 meals per day rather than 2-3 meals as it has been found in recent research that eating in small amounts with more intervals is the better way which not only helps you in keeping full for a longer period, but is also a fundamental technique to lose weight.

Shilpa Shetty Kundra; an Indian actress had admitted herself that she used to have fox-nuts post-pregnancy and it helped her in shedding a considerable amount of post-pregnancy weight.

I also want to share my own experience; I used to weigh 74kgs post-pregnancy and I made sure that whenever I feel hungry for snacks or namkeens, I had fox-nuts. Within one year of my delivery, I shredded those extra kgs and turned out to be in better shape than ever.

Fox-nuts/makhana/lotus seed is believed to be one of the super foods in the post-pregnancy diet. Lotus seeds, i.e. makhanas, are rich in Vitamin B complexes and fiber, which not only helps in burning calories but also lowers the glucose levels in your blood. Besides, they are amazing super foods that help in increasing the milk supply in new mothers and aid weight loss. So if I can do that so effortlessly; losing almost 20kgs post pregnancy, then why can't you?

Working out is the only solution

I still remember the moment I was preparing for a pageant and I wanted to reduce 1-1.5 inches from my waist. The competition was 20 days long and my inches were not reducing despite doing a hardcore workout. I consulted a nutritionist, and she asked me to change my diet a little bit. And you won't believe that in 10 days, I reduced 2kg of weight and a few inches.

That indeed played a significant part in me winning the title of Mrs. Delhi NCR 2018 and it also boosted my career in modeling. It was also the reason I decided to excel in the field of nutrition; diet indeed plays a significant role in the fitness routine.

I remember when my baby was one year old; I was lactating, leaving hardly any time to go to the gym. However, I still managed to lose 20kgs of weight just by planning my diets according to my goals and my nutritional requirements.

It is essential to understand that the food we eat plays a major role in maintaining our fitness. Not everybody on this planet can lift the weights as some are busy with work, some have joints issues, sometimes the gym is not available everywhere and many more reasons.

According to a study, about 80% of gym memberships go unused. It is said that "you can't out-exercise a bad diet," and this is the bottom line when it comes to maintaining a healthy body. There must always be the 80 /20 percent fitness rule, which means; give 80% importance to nutrition and 20% to exercise.

Say NO to Cravings during Diet Plans

I love chocolates, so I always have dark chocolates in my refrigerator. I love to have sweets, so I always have dry fruits and jaggery bars in my kitchen. I love to eat sandwiches, so I make it myself at home with whole grain bread, giving it a healthy twist.

The point is; I eat whatever I crave for but giving it a healthy flair. Besides, there are days when I eat pizzas from Dominos, burgers from McD and Hot dogs from SubWay as a part of my Cheat days. On my weight loss journey, I always made sure that I have dark chocolates, yoghurt and jaggery cubes in my kitchen to satisfy my cravings for sweets. I have a sweet tooth, so I ensure to choose healthy stuffs.

There is a way to satisfy your cravings by swapping to healthy alternatives; like switching ice-cream for sorbet, pina colada for a mojito, milk chocolate for dark chocolate, hard candy for frozen grapes, butter for avocado or peanut butter, sugar for jaggery and many more.

Food cravings cause irresistible urges to eat and are intense. The foods which are high in sugars or other carbohydrates cause cravings, and are difficult to control. So eating healthily doesn't mean you have to give up on your favorite foods and cravings, it's just about the food choices we make.

While on a diet journey, you can often plan a cheat meal for yourself so that it can satisfy your hunger for cravings. I have included a separate chapter on cheat meals so that you can also learn to plan for them while preparing the diet plans. I always recommend planning a new diet plan every week to make your diet free from monotony.

Diet Means Low Energy All Day

I on my weight loss journey never felt out of energy or fatigue despite being lactating. Rather, I used to do chores, play with my baby all day, taking her for walks and I still felt more energetic than before. If you set up your diet properly with well-defined goals, then you will enjoy this journey.

In 2011, Novak Djokovic had what sportswriters called the 'greatest single season' ever by a professional tennis player; he won ten titles, three Grand Slams, and forty-three consecutive matches. Remarkably, less than two years earlier, this champion could barely complete a tournament.

How did a player who was once plagued by aches, breathing difficulties, and injuries on the court suddenly become the no.1 ranked tennis player in the world?

The answer is astonishing; he changed what he ate. Novak djkovic wrote in his book "SERVE TO WIN" about how changes in his diet helped him become the world no. 1 Tennis player. I strongly recommend reading this book for those who have any doubts regarding healthy eating.

A properly planned diet makes you more active rather than causing fatigue. The energy in our body totally depends on the kind of food we eat. Eating healthy food swaps can boost up your metabolism and keep you more active as compared to junk and oily food which causes laziness and procrastination.

Diet is Expensive

While I was on my weight loss journey, I used to plan my meals in a way I can use the seasonal fruits, vegetables and things that were already present in my kitchen. So I figured out that during all this my expenditure was much less than before.

If you are aiming to lose weight, then it can be done effectively from the products available in your kitchen without buying any expensive supplements. Planning your meals for the week will allow you to buy only what you're sure you will use by checking out what you already have in your cupboards first.

While planning your meals, choose the options you can cook by yourself so that you won't need to buy anything extra, hence saving a lot of money. Always try to buy whole foods as they are often less expensive than their processed counterpart and offer more nutrients.

By the end of this book, I'll be sharing a list of some super foods which are present in every household and are of great nutritional value; they will help you in losing weight more effectively as compared to those expensive supplements. With this, you will also give up on your bad food habits and ultimately save a lot of money.

Diet Plans are Only for Weight Loss

A Bollywood actor, Aamir Khan had to gain weight to play wrestler Mahavir Phogat in his movie, Dangal; he lost all those kilograms to play a younger version. And he has done a fabulous job of gaining around 25kg for the second phase of shooting for Dangal. But how did he manage all that in such a short time? The key is a balanced diet.

Diet plans are not only for those who want to lose weight; rather, they are for everyone. Yes, I mean every single individual needs to have a planned and balanced diet, even to maintain. For example; initially when I was losing weight, I planned my diet accordingly, opted for foods which aid in weight loss and after losing fat, I switched my diet from weight loss diet to muscle gaining diet. So this is how it works.

By the end of this book, you will be able to plan your diet according to your goal, be it gaining weight, losing weight or maintaining a healthy weight.

Lost Weight Comes Back Once You Stop Your Diet

Rahul, one of my client who lost 12kgs and came down from 80 to 68kgs is maintaining this healthy weight since a year because when he started the journey, he aimed for a long term goal of changing his poor eating habits, changing his lifestyle and yes he partied every weekend, but now, he knows what the healthy food swaps are and even if he is eating unhealthily, he knows how much amount to consume.

I will also like to give the example of myself as I've been maintaining my weight for the past ten months because I have changed my eating habits and lifestyle. After the end of every diet, people put on weight because they stop putting the same amount of work into maintaining weight as they did to lose it in the first place.

This happens when you are aimed at temporary weight loss and once you achieve your target, you get back to your old lifestyle. But if you know the amount of calories you need to consume to maintain the weight, you can never gain it back.

One hack I'll tell you; measure your weight every day so that it will daily remind you the amount of effort you put in for the weight and automatically, your subconscious mind will always tell you that you have to maintain your weight. Surround yourself with reminders of what living a healthy life means. Thus weight, once lost by your healthy eating habits, will remain forever.

Summary

Always remember that diet plans can be for anyone and not necessarily for the person who wants to lose weight. Diet doesn't mean starving, buying expensive foods or supplements, or you can't lose weight if you have some medical history or if you are ageing.

Diet plan simply means eating according to our bodies' nutritional requirements in a more balanced way, and thus aiming at changing your lifestyle.

In the next chapter, we will see why is it important to lose weight or look fit.

Chapter Two – Why is it Important to Shed those Extra KGS?

"When it comes to eating right and exercising, there is no 'I'll start tomorrow.' Tomorrow is a disease"-**V.L. Allinear**.

One of my uncles who used to be a great time foodie and used to say "enjoy your life and eat whatever you want to eat, nothing will happen", was diagnosed with diabetes a few months back. It created a lot of stress among the family members and the people who are attached to him.

Every one of us at some point in time wonder that life is given to us once, so why not live freely and eat whatever you feel like? It is just that you are not aware of the fact of how your lifestyle can have an irreversible impact on your health.

It's necessary to maintain a healthy lifestyle if you want to have a disease-free life. So, here in this chapter, we will discuss why it is crucial to lose weight. Does your health have any effect on your life chances, achievements, aspirations or the people surrounding you?

Avenues of Success Are Wide

What do you think; with whom will your boss get impressed? A fit and healthy man, full of confidence, very smartly dressed, looks young, always full of energy OR a man who has poor eating habits, low confidence, bulges that can be seen clearly in attire, low in energy as well as in confidence? I think the first one impressed us all.

Yes, your outlook can indeed impact your avenues of success both in negative as well as positive ways. It is said that a healthy and fit person always seems to be full of confidence as compared to a man who is lacking in fitness. So it is essential to maintain your healthy weight as you never know which opportunity is knocking at your door.

The overweight and body fat stops you from doing many things like not wanting to be a part of any sport or any activity that requires strength and stamina. The extra kgs in your body and your poor lifestyle can surely be a symptom of any big disease in future. To avoid this condition, it is indispensable to keep an eye on your body's nutritional requirements. If you have a sedentary lifestyle, you need to either make it a little active or plan your diet accordingly. Early diet plans are in anyway better than pills. If you look fit, healthy and have a good lifestyle, then your boss will show more confidence in you, gives you more projects because fitness is the first step to success.

For example, one of my clients who faced multiple rejections in interviews talked to me. In our conversations, we figured out that he was not confident about his body which may be one of the reasons of getting fewer marks in interviews. So I recommended some minor changes in his eating habits and the results were so good that he got in better shape with weight loss and he felt more confident, which helped him to perform better and fetched him a job of his choice.

Be an Inspiration

When I gained weight post-pregnancy, my confidence dropped down and I kept thinking all day that modeling was a history for me as I never hoped to get back into the industry with those bulges. When I started my fat loss journey a few months later while following my diet plans, I got back to a better shape than ever and everyone around me was surprised to see my transformation; those who were pregnant found a new ray of hope that when I could, then they can also get back to shape; those who lost hope, gained back the motivation to start their fat loss journey.

It is important to shed those extra kgs so that the people around you can get inspired by you, and you can be a motivation for them. So yes, it depends on you how you want the society to look at you.

Our children follow our footsteps, so it is most likely that if you have a poor health and lifestyle, your children will also have the same. It must have happened to you that you see someone lost his weight in a short time and you suddenly get inspired to get away with your bulges and start doing gym or Zumba to get the results. But within a few days, that motivation goes away and you end up wasting your hard-earned money on these activities.

If this has ever happened to you, then you have the right book in your hands. By the end of this book, you will be able to plan your diet and start getting results way faster than other methods. Just like you got inspired by other people, there will be a time very soon, when people will get inspired by you.

It is truly said that "it is never too late for good beginnings"; be fit, smart and confident, and the people around you will admire you, look upon you, and will make you the ideal. And what more is there to life? It gives me so much satisfaction when people text me that "I want to look like you"; nothing in life can beat that happiness and contentment.

Centre of Attraction

After having a baby and shedding that pregnancy weight, I attended a few get-togethers. Some friends couldn't believe that I am a mother of a 1.5 yrs old girl so they came running to me, asking for tips and tricks that helped me in my transformation, and it always feels good when you can hold someone's attraction.

How does it feel when you attend someone's wedding or party and you prepared hard for it but nobody appreciates you or pays attention to you? Or let's take it this way; you bought a good expensive branded dress for a party and your friend just wore a casual outfit. Yet, she looked attractive because she is fit while your bulges made even an expensive dress look average on you.

Fitness is the thing that gives you appreciation everywhere and holds people attention on you. Another advantage of a fit and healthy body is that you can fit in any old clothes, your favorite prom-nightdress, and you will have many options rather than opting for choices that will cover your entire body to hide those bulges. A fit and healthy individual looks younger in age and more energetic, and always on his/her toes to do any work.

Gain Confidence

What is the first thing you notice in a group photograph of you and your friends? Isn't it yourself, your appearance or whether your pose in the picture makes you look slim? And if by chance your bulges are visible in the photograph or you are looking fat than everyone, the first thing you wish is that it doesn't get posted on social media.

Your fit and healthy body is directly proportional to your confidence. It has been seen in schools and colleges; fat individuals often get bullied; they are called by funny names which is disheartening for them. If your lifestyle and your eating habits are the reasons behind your fat and weight gain, then you should give yourself a wake-up call as soon as possible. Remember, it's never too late for good beginnings because your fitness will be an answer.

What happens when you transform yourself from fat to fab? People will admire you, and suddenly you will notice that you have become more confident than before, your inputs in your office or business will escalate, and you will discover the new YOU.

For example; one of my clients, Radhika was very fit but suddenly, she got a transfer to a new place that changed her lifestyle and eating habits which includes most of the junk foods and drinks. After some months when she came back for a home visit, all the people who knew her noticed that she had gained some serious weight; she couldn't fit in her old clothes, and when she measured her weight, it was 7kgs more than she used to weigh usually.

The girl who used to be very confident about her looks now looked tensed and wanted to lose those extra kgs. So, I planned a diet for her so that she can eat everything but smartly as she had to attend office parties and get-togethers. With this diet, she effortlessly lost some serious weight and gained her confidence back.

Losing weight will not only give you confidence, but will also make you more appealing and young forever.

Say Goodbye to Body-Shaming

How would you feel to be addressed as mota or moti in front of anyone? Do you feel humiliated? This is the reality of society.

As quoted by Sandra Amodt in her book *"The Unintended Consequences of Our Obsession with Weight Loss"*, Children and teenagers are especially vulnerable to fat-shaming; a study of 2,500 American girls who were fat-shamed found that these girls were twice likely to gain weight within the next five years than those who weren't criticized about their weight. We people don't see an individual for his/her sense of humor, intelligence, and personality, but their body. I have come across people who have been body-shamed and want to lose weight quickly.

If this body-shaming is happening with you just because you are having unhealthy food and you seriously want to avoid that, you must learn how to plan your diets. But do it only when you are doing it for yourself, or your inner voice makes you do so.

For example; regarding my weight loss journey, many of my dear ones questioned why I lost weight. They said "you were looking good like that" and I always reply them that "maybe I was looking good to you, but I was not comfortable in that body", and so thereby, I shed those extra kgs. Call for maintaining your body must come from your inner self rather than the societal pressures.

Feel Energetic and Young All the Time

We all have that one friend who is a workaholic and remains active throughout the day. Remember those friends in college or your colleagues who after study or office don't miss sports. You must be wondering about the secret of their energy. There is only one secret that is there to a healthy body; if you are suffering from laziness and procrastination, the fault lies in your lifestyle.

According to a report by World Health Organization (WHO), People in poor health are less likely to work and when in work, are less productive to get good health. People should follow a healthy lifestyle; people who are not involved in the healthy lifestyle may suffer a range of health disorders like overweight, high blood pressure, heart disease, obesity, diabetes, high cholesterol, kidney problems, liver disorders and so many.

An unhealthy body gets tired very quickly and a tired body easily loses motivation and self-confidence. Nowadays, we are so much dependent on the outside junk food that we don't want to have homemade food. There is no problem eating outside food; occasionally, the problem starts when it becomes your addiction.

Junk foods are the foods that contribute a lot of calories with little nutritional value; they are also low in satiation value, i.e. people don't tend to feel full when they eat them which lead to overeating. There are a lot of things related to junk food and not only calories; the hygiene issues plus the chemicals that are used to lure your taste buds and the usage of processed foods in making them.

All these lead to fat gain and other health issues such as cholesterol issues, and this makes our body less energetic and lazy, and we begin to age much earlier, though it does not mean that one should altogether avoid eating junk food. It is always better to eat homemade stuff as it adds to your skills and you know the amount and kinds of ingredients you are using.

You can also improvise them by keeping some healthy side of it.

For example; I always recommend a diet that focuses more on homemade food with healthy ingredients and some clients are also baking their loaves of bread as they love it more than the bakery ones; they can add the healthy seeds and nuts to it while using healthy flours rather than refined flours. Our food choices directly have an impact on our energy levels and our looks. So to look young and energetic, it's never too late to opt for healthy food swaps.

Summary

In this chapter, we discussed why it is essential to maintain a healthy body. Whether it is the new avenues of success or you want to be an inspiration for all, be a centre of attraction or want to be disease-free etc. Only your food can give you a healthy body or can result in a diseased body; the choice is yours. Remember the more you remain fit, the more confident and energetic you are.

In the next chapter, well be discussing how you can lose weight. We will be learning about the different ways and techniques.

Chapter Three– How to Lose Weight

"You didn't gain all your weight in one day; you won't lose it in one day. Be patient with yourself"- **Jenna Wolfe.**

According to a study, it has been found that obesity and overweight are considered to be the fifth cause of death all over the world. In 2008, the number of overweight adults was 1.5 billion of which 200 million of them were obese men and nearly 300 million were obese women.

This chapter deals with the various methods used all over the world and will help you to lose extra inches. While losing weight, you must also give adequate attention to the approach you are opting for. Most often, people follow the method used by their known ones to lose weight without knowing whether the same approach will work for them the same way.

The approach that may work for me to lose weight may not work for you. That's why it is essential for you to learn the method that suits you well.

Gymnasium

My husband has paid several annual memberships of gym thinking that this will force him to be regular in the gym, but the story continues hardly for 10-15 days and then as usual, procrastination and laziness overcomes motivation.

According to a study, about 80% of gym memberships go unused. You might have heard or experienced yourself that once you pay the annual fee of the gym, then you do the gym just for a few days which means money gets wasted along with your efforts, and you end up with the same weight.

The gym should be used only if you are aiming at strength building or you want to participate in some bodybuilding competition. Even the gym instructors also recommend following a proper diet plan if you want to build muscles. Diet is not only for those who are aiming at weight loss, but also for those who want to build abs or build muscles.

Moreover, if you have back problems, knee joints issues or a doctor advised you to avoid heavy exercises, then it is better to avoid the gym so as not to aggravate the problem. In such cases, what works for you is a healthy diet plan. This book is not only for those who want to lose weight, it will also help you to plan your diet if you want to build muscles or maintain a healthy weight.

Yoga

Shilpa Shetty Kundra swears by yoga and has always promoted it saying that it keeps her fit and that hourglass figure of hers is perfect all the time. But she has always said in her interviews that along with yoga, it is the healthy diet that keeps her fit even at the age of 45.

Yoga is an effective tool if you want to lose weight. But more than this, the practice of yoga supports the physical, mental, and spiritual development that allows you to create the best version of yourself. Yoga focuses more on mindfulness which makes you conscious of the foods that affect your body, mind and spirit.

Though it helps in the calmness of mind and results in better sleep which is a significant factor for losing weight, it is also a choice for people who are more drawn towards spirituality and peace of mind. But again, I have seen consistency issues in people; some find it boring and while others don't have the patience.

A proper healthy diet is a must in any kind of exercise we do because our body reacts according to the fuel we put in it.

Outdoor Activity

Bollywood celebrities such as John Abraham, Rahul Bose, and Milind Soman like running marathons to keep themselves fit. Running and jogging have immense health benefits; they help in building strong bones, strengthening muscles, improving cardiovascular fitness and maintaining a healthy weight. Despite all its benefits, running without a proper guidance can affect you negatively. I have seen people running too much, putting themselves under stress, impacting their hormones and decreasing their abilities to lose fat.

The increase in air pollution in urban areas has put runners' health at risk. Even wearing of masks is not recommended while working out as it affects the lungs. If you are walking or running few times a week, it is always recommended that you focus on your eating habit; this is because eating according to your body's nutritional requirement, tracking your daily calorie intake and planning a healthy diet for yourself will keep your body enriched with vitamins and minerals, and thus keeping diseases away.

One of the problems most of the runners face these days is the absence of tracks which often results in early age knee problem. Studies have shown that running too much on cardio machines also impact your knees. However, everyday walking for a few minutes is always recommended even if you are only following diet approach to reach your goals.

Swimming

One of my friends works in MNC and is settled in UK. Due to his sedentary lifestyle and physically inactive schedule, he gained around 20kgs. A few months back, we came in contact and he told me he has to lose some weight and I asked him to go swim with his friends.

For two months now, he has been regular and spends 20-40 min in this exercise. And along with this, he has promised to change his food habits which used to be mostly junk and processed foods. And within2 months he lost around 10kgs and he is overwhelmed with his changed lifestyle and good eating habits.

It is found according to a study that most of the people who want to lose weight see swimming as a better option. Swimming does not only provide you with relief from hot temperature, it is also an enjoyable activity you can enjoy with family.

Swimming helps in losing weight and toning your body. If you are aiming to lose that belly fat, it is advisable to swim early in the morning so that the fat stored in the body can be utilized as energy. Swimming involves a full-body workout. While at the start, you should swim slowly and then keep on increasing your pace. Swimming for 4-5 days a week is enough to lose fat. If you have any back problem or any joint issue, then it is always advised to consult a doctor first as swimming involves the entire muscles workout which can aggravate your pain. With any weight loss program, you burn more calories than you take in, so adjustments in your diet are always required.

One must keep in mind that swimming may cause the appetite to increase substantially, thus taking more vegetables, protein shakes and healthy food is always recommended than snacking on junk foods.

Cycling

Sonakshi Sinha, a famous Bollywood actress, has lost 30kgs and shaped herself into a slender diva. In her interviews, she told the interviewer that cycling for an hour was one of the many secrets of her transformation. But cycling alone didn't serve the purpose as she has focused on a proper healthy diet as well.

Cycling is a lower-body sport. Even if you are opting for cycling, you necessarily don't need to cycle very hard to lose fat; instead you should go for slow and a long ride to lose your weight. After cycling, it is vital to consume some carbohydrates and proteins. Some people might think that if they eat less or starve themselves, they will lose weight faster. But on the contrary, they will become weak and will face fatigue all the time.

It is necessary that before riding a bike, you need to keep yourself well hydrated; at least two bottles of water intake is highly recommended before riding a bike during hot days. The changing environment, increasing air pollution and especially this pandemic, has put an exceptional condition as it is never recommended to wear a mask while doing exercise as it affects the lungs.

Moreover, you should keep in mind its long term side effects on your health. For instance; according to the Massachusetts Male Aging Study, it was found that in certain circumstances, bike riding can damage nerves and compress arteries in the penis, which may lead to erectile problems due to the reason that seat puts constant pressure on the perineum.

The risk was highest among men who cycled more than three hours a week. If you at all decide to go for cycling or any other physical activity, a balanced diet and proper intake of macronutrients are always considered necessary. This book is aimed at making you self-sufficient to design your meals according to your body's nutritional requirements.

Intermittent Fasting

A Bollywood celebrity, Malaika Arora Khan who has been following intermittent fasting for a year, says that combination of yoga and Intermittent Fasting has been the crucial part of her fitness regime.

You might have heard about intermittent fasting these days; it is very much trending on Social media apps such as Instagram and Facebook. This is nothing but a "time-restricted feeding" and not as tricky as the most common fasting practices. This is also known as the 16/8 method, which is an eating pattern where you cycle between periods of eating and fasting.

One can do the intermittent fasting by skipping the breakfast, eating the first meal at noon and the last meal at 8 pm. So in this way, you are fasting for 16 hours and restricting your eating habits to 8-hour window. It does not require you to eat any specific food; rather, it doesn't talk about the foods to eat and focuses more on when you should eat them.

This method focuses on splitting the week or day into eating periods and fasting periods. At the start, you may face difficulty but in the end, you will feel better and more energetic. It is not recommended to eat any food during the fasting period, although you can have low caloric beverages like tea, coffee and water. In the past, we humans tend to do fasting to allow our body to thrive in famine; thus, it is naturally inbuilt in humans.

Fasting also helps cellular repair processes and helps in lowering blood sugar and insulin levels. But this method is not for everyone. For example; people having a history of an eating disorder or suffering from diabetes and hyperglycemia, or the people feeling nauseous without eating for long etc. should avoid this approach.

According to a study, if energy and protein are excessively restricted, there's a real risk of nutrient deficiencies, electrolyte abnormalities, and fertility and reproductive issues in women. So it is imperative to know about your body, and then choose the method for losing weight.

Healthy Eating

All the Bollywood music lovers must be aware of Adnan Sami, one of the Bollywood singers and music composers. In his earlier days, he weighed 230kg, but now his transformation to 75kg has amazed everyone. How would he have done that? The secret is a healthy diet.

Being overweight, he couldn't do gym and other workout programs so all he followed was a strict diet plan; giving up on bread, junk foods, and white rice from his meals. He also ensured that he has a regular walk for a few minutes each day without failure.

Healthy eating coupled with moderate walking or exercise can do miracles for anyone at any age. Our eating habits matter a lot and play a significant role in losing fat and staying away from diseases. As said by Dr. Alan Christianson in his book; *"The Metabolism Reset Diet"* that our modern, high-intake, heavily processed diets place a lot of stress on our livers. They tend to get clogged with wastes that prevent them from processing energy efficiently.

These days, people are relying more on junk food due to several reasons and I agree that it's luring, but once you understand its long term consequences on your health, you will want to avoid this as much as possible. You must always keep in mind that processed foods are a big NO if you are aiming for a healthy body.

Processed meals and sugar provide little to no benefit, and they make you fat, sluggish and weak as they've been chemically altered. They make you want to eat more without satisfying your cravings and hunger. As quoted by Dave Asprey in his book *"Bulletproof Diet"*, Monosodium glutamate or MSG is the most common artificial flavor used in processed foods. MSG causes your cells to send signals to each other, so they become activated and overexcited. And when your cells die or get damaged, your brain sends signals requesting more energy, which triggers a headache, mood swings or craving for sweets – the fastest sources of energy.

For example; on my weight loss journey, I ate everything from stuffed parantha to subs, but all are homemade. All I did was replaced some of my foods with their better alternatives such as mayonnaise with mustard sauce, refined oil to ghee/ coconut oil/olive oil, white rice to brown rice, regular bread to multigrain bread, butter to peanut butter or white butter and so on.

Having a perfect diet plan is today's need, and one myth you have to throw out of your mind is that dieting doesn't mean starving or eating less; it's like eating tastier, healthier and more variety of food, more frequently like 5-6 meals per day rather than3 meals per day in a balanced way according to your nutritional requirements.

One important thing which you must keep in your mind is your calorie count; the amount of calorie consumption and macronutrients your body needs and eating according to it. If someone is asking you to opt for supplements or pills to lose weight, then you are talking to the wrong person.

You can lose weight from the ingredients of your kitchen, you only need to be little aware of their benefits which I promise to deliver through this book. There are various kinds of a diet that you can follow according to your preference which will be explained in the forthcoming chapter.

Summary

In this chapter, you learned about the various methods that can help you to lose weights such as going to gym, running, swimming, yoga, intermittent fasting and dieting. You have to choose the right approach that suits your body deliberately. Each approach has its pros and cons.

Whatever path you take, it is always recommended to incorporate healthy dieting in it for better, faster and long-lasting results. Even if you rely only on healthy eating approach, the results are guaranteed.

In the next chapter, you will learn about the various kinds of diet in the world to make you chose your diet rationally. So stay alert, this is the most exciting part.

PART II - Planning Your Diet like an Expert in Five Steps

Chapter Four – STEP I (Understanding Different Types of Diets)

"Your diet is a bank account; good food choices are good investments"- **Bethany Frankel.**

Since you are in the process of learning to plan your diet, it is imperative to know what diet means. How many types of diets are there; the foods that need to be eaten or avoided in a particular diet? What are its good and bad impacts on our health while choosing a specific diet?

In nutrition, diet is the sum of foods consumed by a person. It implies the use of a specific intake of nutrition for health or weight-management reasons. There are various kinds of diets practiced around the world. The type of diet you choose depends upon your food choices, i.e. whether you are a vegetarian or non-vegetarian, the availability of food suits your health.

Any diet can be chosen either to lose weight or gain weight. When a person tends to go on a diet, it may balance his/her energy level and increase or decrease the fats stored by the body.

If you are overweight or obese, changing to a diet and lifestyle that allows you to burn more calories than you consume may improve your overall health and prevent the diseases that are attributed in part to weight such as heart disease and diabetes. If a person is underweight due to illness or malnutrition, he may change his diet to promote weight gain.

There are five significant diet types all across the world. They include:

1. Paleo Diet
2. Ketogenic Diet
3. Indian Diet
4. Mediterranean Diet
5. Vegan Diet

We will discuss each of these in detail, to make you capable of choosing the best one for yourself.

1. Paleo Diet

The famous American singer, Miley Cyrus had been suffering from an eating disorder in the past. To improve her eating habits, she has gone Paleo dieting with emphasizes on gluten-free products. She, in one of her interviews, accepted that due the changes in her diet, she feels great with her skin and physical appearance; and mental health is fantastic after the diet.

Paleo diet mimics our hunters and gatherers, i.e. anything that can be hunted or gathered is allowed to be eaten in this diet, abandoning the entire sugar intake. The only sugar that can be consumed is through fruits. In the Paleo diet, dairy products are also prohibited. The paleo diet contains a fewer number of carbohydrates which will lead to a decreased amount of glucose. So your body system will then begin to use fat as its fuel source, leading to fat loss.

While choosing this diet, the foods that may be consumed are given below.

What can you eat?

- Grass-fed meat; beef, chicken, pork, turkey
- Eggs(Pasteurized)
- Fish
- Vegetables and fruits
- Nuts and seeds
- Tubers and yams

- Extra virgin Olive oil, Coconut oil, Avocado oil
- Himalayan salt, Sea salt, Turmeric, Ginger, Garlic etc

What can you not eat?

- Any processed foods
- Sugar; Candy, Donuts, Pastries, Soft drinks, Table Sugar, Ice-creams
- Grains; Oats, Barley, Pasta, Wheat, Rye
- Dairy
- Factory Animals
- Vegetable Oils
- Trans-fats
- Legumes
- Anything that comes in a wrapper or a box etc

By this list of foods, you now have a fair idea about what kind of diet Paleo is. This diet is beneficial if you have Type-2 diabetes. It also helps in reducing inflammation and digestive stress and has been proven highly beneficial for weight loss. But it has been observed by the people following this diet that it gets very restricted. It becomes a real challenge if you are a vegan, and can get expensive for you due to the food choices it offers.

2. Ketogenic Diet

You must have heard about or seen the miraculous weight loss transformation of Anant Ambani, son of Mukesh Ambani. He lost 108kgs of weight in just 18 months without any weight loss surgery. Apart from exercises, diet played a significant role in his transformation.

Being born with asthma and diabetes, it was not an easy journey for him as he also had to take care of the food choices that work for him the best. He adopted a ketogenic diet which involves a low carb diet with adequate fat and protein, and since he was a diabetic, he had to keep himself stuck to zero sugar intake.

The ketogenic diet is a low carb and high-fat diet. It aims at drastically reducing carbohydrates intake and focuses on eating more calories from fat. Lack of carbohydrates put your body in a metabolic state called ketosis. When this happens, your body starts burning fats for energy and thus turns fat into ketones in the liver and therefore supplies energy to the brain.

Ketones are the compounds that are created from fats in the liver, and since the world is overloaded with refined carbohydrates, our bodies are in the habit of using glucose as energy for all its needs. If you follow this diet, then for some initial days, you may experience keto flu that may lead to digestive discomfort, headaches and a feeling of nausea and fatigue. But after this flu, your body will start burning fats and you'll feel better and start to lose weight in the process.

What can you eat in a ketogenic diet?

- Meats
- Fatty Fish
- Eggs
- Butter and Cream
- Cheese
- Nuts and Seeds
- Healthy Oils
- Avocados
- Vegetables etc

What can you not eat or need to avoid?

- Any processed foods
- Sugar; Candy, Donuts, Pastries, Soft drinks, Table sugars, Ice creams
- Grains; Oats, Barley, Pasta, Wheat, Rye
- Dairy Products
- Fruits
- Factory Animals
- Vegetable Oils
- Trans-fats
- Legumes
- Anything that comes in a wrapper or a box etc

So this is the list of what you can and cannot eat in this diet. There are a few advantages of this diet such as; you lose some serious weight and it is also recommended for people who have Type-2 diabetes. It also helps in reducing the risk of cancer and Alzheimer disease. But it is very restricted as far as food choices are concerned. Sometimes while following this diet, you may experience loss of muscle mass which may lead to low energy levels for the workout.

The ketogenic diet is found to be useful for people who are overweight, diabetic or looking to improve their metabolic health. At the same time, it is considered less suitable for elite athletes and people who wish to add muscle or weight.

3. Indian diet

Most of the people aiming for weight loss think that to lose weight, they have to try modern diets, leaving their roots. But one thing I would like to mention is that this is purely a misconception. It is much easier to lose diet with the food you have been eating since childhood. Take myself for an example; I on my weight loss journey stuck to the Indian diet, and yet managed to lose 20kgs in 5 months. It is not necessary to try fancy diets, what you have to take care of are the number of calories and the macronutrients intake.

Indian diet is one of the most balanced diets as it is loaded with proteins, carbohydrates, fats and fibers. It includes some nutritious foods such as grains, lentils, healthy fats, vegetables and fruits. Most people have a misconception that a weight loss diet requires drastic changes in diet such as intermittent fasting, 10-week diet, keto diet or health supplements. You just need a balanced diet with the right proportions of all food groups.

There are many ways to cook Indian food by adding varieties in your foods, and if you cook them healthily, it may taste even better. Also, many Indian traditional spices and herbs are incredibly healthy such as chilies, turmeric, garlic, cinnamon, cardamom, ginger and basil leaves; if appropriately added to your food.

Fruits and vegetables such as spinach, okra, tomato, mushroom, cabbage, apple, guava, pomegranate, etc. provides an adequate amount of vitamins and nutrients in this diet. Kidney beans, chickpeas and other legumes such a mug bean, black-eyed pea, lentils and pulses are an essential part of Indian diet and are also a good source of proteins. Dairy products form an integral part of Indian meals such as milk, cheese, buttermilk tofu, curd, ghee etc.

What can you eat?

- Grains; wheat and barley
- Rice
- Lentils
- Fruits and vegetables
- Dairy products; buttermilk, yoghurt
- Chicken/lamb etc

What do you need to avoid?

- Any processed foods
- Sugar; candy, doughnuts, pastries, soft drinks, table sugar, ice creams
- Refined grains
- Vegetable oils
- Trans-fats etc

Indian diets are highly skewed towards high carbs. For example; a medium bowl of Dal has 17gms of proteins but 40gms of carbs. Similarly, chapatti has fewer proteins and more carbs. Apart from this, it is suitable for people suffering from heart diseases, stroke and other chronic ailments; it helps in reducing inflammation and being balanced in nutrition. It satisfies hunger and cravings.

4. Mediterranean Diet

This diet is quite popular among Hollywood stars. You must know about Spanish actress, Penelope Cruz who was spotted saying in an interview that it is the

Mediterranean diet that helps her to keep fit and healthy. She gives all the credits to this diet for coming back in shape in just four months after delivering her baby boy. Apart from her, many celebrities are in awe of this diet such as Lady Gaga, Robert de Niro and many more.

This diet is inspired by eating habits of Greece, Spain, Southern Italy, in the 1940s and 1950s.The principle of this diet is proportionally high consumption of olive oils, legumes, unrefined sugars. This diet has high quantities of fruits and vegetables, which is grossly missing in many diets around the world. It also contains moderate to increased consumption of fish, dairy products, wine and low consumption of red meat products. Healthy fats are the mainstay of Mediterranean diets like usage of olive oils, which provides monounsaturated fat and has been found to lower total cholesterol and low-density lipoprotein (LDL or "bad") cholesterol levels. Usage of fatty fish in the Mediterranean diet makes the foods rich in omega-3 fatty acids and helps in reducing the inflammation in the body. Thus, it is also considered to be a heart-friendly diet.

What can you eat?

- Vegetable and fruits
- Nuts and seeds
- Legumes
- Whole grains
- Bread
- Fish and other kinds of seafood
- Extra-virgin olive oil
- Herbs and spices
- Poultry eggs: cheese and yoghurt etc

What do you need to avoid?

- Any processed food
- Sugar; candy, donuts, pastries, soft drinks, table sugar, ice- creams
- Refined grains
- Dairy
- Factory animals
- Vegetable oils
- Trans-fats
- Anything that comes in a wrapper or box etc

In this diet, vitamins and minerals are very high, which helps in fighting against free radicals. This kind of diet also reduces the risk of heart diseases, stroke, and other chronic ailments. It is strongly recommended for people suffering from type-2 diabetes.

While following this diet, if you overdo the calories when it comes to wine, olive oil and bread, it may result in fat gain. However, if you monitor your calorie intake and eating habits, then this can prove to be the best diet.

5. Vegan Diet

I remember reading the interview of a famous Indian cricketer, Virat Kohli who adopted vegan in October 2018 as he went through a major fitness transformation. He decided to give up on animal-based products. The changes in his food habit did improve not only his fitness but also his game.

Veganism in a strict sense is a process which excludes all the animal-based products, including honey as honeybees produce it. This kind of diet has become very popular these days due to increasing inclination of people towards ethical, environmental, health and social reasons. This diet has various health benefits but lacks in total nutritional requirements of your body. A vegan diet helps in controlling blood sugar levels and also keeps type-2 diabetes at bay. Vegan diets are also effective at reducing total cholesterol.

What can you eat?

- All fruits and vegetables
- Grains; wheat, rye, and barley
- Beans and legumes
- Nuts and seeds
- Coconut oil, avocado oil
- Tubers and yams

What do you need to avoid?

- All animal foods
- Eggs
- All meats
- Honey
- Dairy and dairy products

However, apart from all the benefits of a vegan diet, there is a drawback that needs to be taken care of. The people following this diet miss out the essential nutrients which are required by the body such as vitamin B12, vitamin D, long-chain omega-3s, iodine, iron, calcium and zinc.

It is not recommended for those with increased requirements, such as children or lactating women. To minimize this deficiency, you can opt for nutrient-rich plant food instead of various processed foods. The use of iron cast pots and pans for cooking are recommended. Avoiding tea or coffee with meals and combining iron-rich foods with a source of vitamin C is beneficial. Few tips and tricks can help you to reach your nutritional requirements in this diet.

Summary

In this chapter, we learned about the different types of diets, their impacts on health. It is for you to identify which diet is best suited according to your food choices. Every diet has its pros and cons, but the critical point is to know how it will benefit our body in longer terms.

If you want a heart-healthy diet, you can opt for the Mediterranean. If you wish to be on a vegetarian side, then the vegan diet is the best, and if you want those north Indian delicacies in your weight loss journey, you can go for Indian diet, and so on.

In the next chapter, we will learn about specific components, methods and formulas of our TDEE and BMR, which forms the basis of meal planning.

Chapter Five - STEP II (Know Your Body and Its Requirements)

I remember when my sister and I were in college, I used to complain to my mother why my sister couldn't get fat despite eating all day. Yes, my sister used to have all the delicacies she could have, but it never added fat to her body. While anyone who meets me always called me chubby, I used to feel so bad that despite eating very little, why I put on weight so fast?

So, all my youthful days went on by me making food choices that wouldn't make me fat. But later, I realized that it is all about metabolism; my sister had a perfect metabolism, so I focused on working on it.

I studied a lot about metabolism and followed advices of health experts because of which, now I can say "yes I have a healthy metabolism". You must have heard people saying that his/her metabolism is excellent while some people are complaining of low metabolism.

What is meant by metabolism, and how does it affect your body?

Metabolism involves all the chemical reactions that the body needs to function. Metabolism is linked to nutrition. Most fad diets promote unhealthy, short-term weight loss by restricting the fuel and nutrients that your body needs. These diets are counterproductive because they often exacerbate the core problem– your metabolism. Diet planning is essential for good metabolism and to satisfy our nutritional requirements. While planning any diet, you should always take care of some metrics to figure your baseline, i.e. TDEE (Total daily energy expenditure).

TDEE is generally the maintenance of calorie intake, i.e. calories you have to consume daily to maintain your body weight. TDEE is just an estimate and not the numbers; therefore, you have to adjust your calorie intake from week to week depending upon the progress you are making, or you are lacking. The most crucial input that TDEE is comprised of is BMR.

Now we will understand BMR, TDEE and their role in diet planning, you can plan your diet precisely according to your body's requirements.

BMR (Basal Metabolic Rate)

You must know about the various functions performed by the body while at rest, which are breathing, repairing cells, blood circulation, developing new cells and many more. Have you ever wondered where the body derives energy to perform these functions? Well, it's nothing except BMR.

BMR is the total energy expressed in calories in which a person needs to keep his body functioning while at rest to maintain the body's essential functions such as breathing, blood circulation, growing and repairing cells. Basal metabolic rate (BMR) affects the rate at which a person burns his calories, resulting in weight gain or weight loss.

The BMR accounts for about 60 to 75% of the daily calorie expenditure by individuals; several factors influence it. Basal Metabolic Rate typically declines by 1–2% per decade after age 20, mostly due to loss of fat-free mass, although it varies from individual to individual.

You can calculate the BMR estimates by knowing the age, sex, weight and height of the person involved using the absolute equations which are given below. If you have more lean muscle mass or more weight, then you tend to have a higher BMR. You can calculate your BMR with several formulas which include:

• The Katch McArdle Equation

BMR= 370+(9.7975* lean mass in pounds)

LEAN MASS= TOTAL WEIGHT – FAT MASS

Example: There is a girl named Sanjana who is 30 years old, her weight is 140 pounds in which her body fat comprises of 30%.

First of all, we will calculate Sanjana's fat mass= 30% of 140 pounds = 42 pounds

Sanjana's lean mass= 140-42= 98 pounds

Sanjana's BMR by The Katch McArdle Equation= 370+ (9.79*98) = 1329.42 calories.

• The Mifflin St. Joer Equation

For Men: BMR = 10* weight (in kgs) + 6.25* height (in cms) - 5* age (in years) + 5

For Women: BMR= 10* weight (in kgs) + 6.25*height (in cms) - 5 * age (in years)– 161

- ## The Harris-Benedict Formula

For Men: BMR= 66 + (13.75 x weight) + (5 x height) – (6.76 x age)

For Women: BMR= 655 + (9.56 x weight) + (1.85 x height) – (4.68 x age)

- ## The Owen formula

For Men: BMR= 879 + (10.2 x weight)

For Women: BMR=795 + (7.2 x weight)

- ## Others

For Men: BMR= 24.2 x weight

For Women: BMR= 22 x weight

However, you need not to worry about these mathematical equations. There is a simple way out for calculating your BMR

> ➤ Simply take your body's weight in pounds and multiply it by 10 (to find approximate readings)
> OR
> ➤ You can know your BMR by using the online calculator. There are various websites, such as calculator.net. You can also search by yourself on Google for different online calculators. You are free to choose any one of them.

TDEE (Total Daily Energy Expenditure)

Once you have estimated your BMR, you just need to multiply this number by an activity multiplier. Activity multipliers depend on the type, intensity, duration, and frequency of physical activity. Energy needs for physical activity may vary from 20% to 70% or more of BMR.

Follow the guidelines below to determine your multiplier:

1. Sedentary (little or no exercise, desk job) = BMR x 1.2
2. Lightly Active (light exercise/sports 1-3 days/week) = BMR x 1.375
3. Moderate Active (moderate exercise/sports 3-5 days/week = BMR x 1.55
4. Very Active (hard exercise/sports 6-7 days/week) = BMR 1.725
5. Extremely Active (hard daily exercise/sport and active physical job OR 2x day training – marathon, contest, etc.) = BMR x 1.9

After multiplying your BMR by your activity multiplier, you have successfully determined your Total Daily Energy Expenditure. Now you can plan your diet according to TDEE while keeping your goals in mind.

Example - there is a girl named Sanjana who is 30 years old; her weight is 140 pounds, her height is 160cms. Her job comprises of a sedentary job, and she goes gym a few times a week.

Multiply weight in pounds by 10 to find BMR and it comes out to be 1400 calories/day.

And if we calculate by an online calculator, it comes out to be 1324 calories/day (slight variations are acceptable between both the methods).

TDEE = [1324 * 1.55] = 2052.2 calories/day (here we multiplied BMR with 1.55 because Sanjana is having a sedentary job with the gym few times a week thus making her moderately active).

TDEE is very important for your diet planning. You have to vary this figure according to your goals, such as:

- Eat equal to or slightly more than TDEE = maintain your current weight, Sanjana has to consume 2052cal to maintain her current weight
- Eat more than TDEE = expect to gain weight, Sanjana has to consume > 2052cal to gain weight
- Eat less than TDEE = expect to lose weight, Sanjana has to consume < 2052cal to lose weight

For now, you just keep this in mind. Sanjana has to eat more than 2052calories to gain her weight and eat less than 2052 calories to lose her weight. But how or how more she has to eat will be discussed further.

Factors that affect metabolism and TDEE

Metabolism and TDEE are essential while planning any diet, and they vary from person to person depending on various factors which are discussed below:

1. **Genetics** – everyone is born different, so some people burn more energy than others and hence, genes play a more significant role in this.

2. **Age** – metabolic rate is highest in fast-growing children but as we reach our 20s and beyond, our metabolic rate gradually slows down due to ageing which changes our activity type and hence everything.

3. **Gender** – men tend to have higher metabolic rates due to a greater level of muscle and lower fat percentage compared to women. And thus we find more fat percentage in women as compared to men.

4. **Bodyweight** – the more you weigh, the higher your metabolic rate will be. Overweight people tend to have higher metabolic rates than leaner individuals due to there being greater overall body mass (muscle and fat) to maintain.

5. **Height** – similar to bodyweight, taller individuals have more overall mass to maintain and therefore higher metabolic rates.

6. **Starvation diets** – the fad diets that induce massive calorie restrictions can cause a massive reduction in metabolic rate as a way to protect against the "famine."

7. **Hormones** – thyroid disorders can cause an increase or decrease in metabolic rate.

8. **Temperature** – increase in both your internal body core temperature and the external temperature of the environment can cause increase in metabolic rate to cool and maintain internal homeostasis.

9. **Exercise** – exercise can increase your metabolic rate, particularly after high-intensity exercise which burns more

calories during Excess Post-Exercise Oxygen Consumption (EPOC).

How TDEE Affects the Meal Plan for Fat Loss Diet or Weight Gain Diet?

So you have your TDEE value with you and now, how you will use that value for fat loss or weight gain diet? Well, whatever your goal is, it is always recommended not to alter these values drastically as it may have reverse effects on your body, just go slow and steady to win the race.

So there are three goals that sought by people to achieve. They are:

1. Lose fat
2. Gain weight
3. Maintain a healthy weight

1. Loose fat

When I say fat loss, I always talk about healthy and sustainable fat loss which amounts to a loss of 1-2lbs (½-1kg) in a week. So if you are aiming for a fat loss diet, then you need to consume [10-30] %

calories<TDEE. For example; if your TDEE says 2000 calories per day, then you should consume [200- 600] <TDEE which amounts between 1400 calories to 1800 calories.

If you are aiming to lose fat faster, then you can opt for the {30% < TDEE}, like you can have 1400 calories/day; otherwise, you can lose the weight enjoying your diet, i.e. {10% < TDEE}, like 1800calories /day. The time your body will take to lose fat will depend on your approach.

But if you try to go beyond 30%, then this can be harmful to your health, and it is more of a starvation diet. For example; trying this 30% fewer calories than your TDEE and if it still does not result in fat loss, although the chances are significantly less, then you should start focusing more on exercise and working rather than reducing your calories to more extent.

The better option is; in the starting, to keep your calorie intake as 30% less than TDEE and observe your control on craving, hunger and then modify accordingly.

2. Gain Weight

If you are trying to gain some weight, you mean you want the muscle gain and not fat gain and thus trying to keep your fat to a minimum level.

For weight gain, I always recommend everyone to try to add 10-15% calories to their TDEE and while keeping some exercise on, it will help them to gain some muscle. One can expect a gain of 1-2 pounds of muscle per month.

For example; if your TDEE is 2000 calories, then you can consume 2200- 2300 calories per day to gain muscle. And remember, muscle gain process is a bit slower than fat loss.

3. Maintaining a healthy weight

For healthy weight management, it is always advisable to consume slightly less than or equal to your TDEE. It will help you with weight management and will avoid the fluctuation of your weight.

For example; if your TDEE is 2000, then you can keep your daily calorie intake around 2000 calories/day for maintaining your current weight.

Summary

In this chapter, we learned about various metrics regarding our metabolism and how we can measure our daily calorie requirements. The BMR formulas involve mathematical calculation and cannot be used smoothly in everyday lives.

An alternative is to use the online BMR calculator, which will require you to fill your age, weight, height and gender. While you plan your diet according to your goals, always keep in mind the calories your body need to lose fat, gain weight or maintain weight and also keeping your macronutrients sufficient.

In the next chapter, we will learn about how to plan your diet.

Chapter Six - STEP III (Creating Your Very Own Perfect Diet Plan)

When the word diet plan comes to your mind, you suddenly think about starving yourself or giving up on your favorite foods. But will that serve your purpose of losing weight or gaining muscles? I have seen people living with this misconception of diet planning.

What does the diet planning mean?

Diet planning doesn't mean starving or eating less; it is just eating the right food in the right quantity and at the right time. Diet planning is crucial if you want to remain fit and healthy. It is the essential thing that one should imbibe in his/ her life, to stay young and disease-free.

In this chapter, you will learn about how you can plan your diet without any external help, the steps you should keep in mind while preparing your diet, and thus you can become your own diet planner. The goal is to have nutritionally adequate diets and to ensure that the probability of nutrient inadequacy or excess is acceptably low.

Six Principles

There are six principles which are essential to incorporate in any diet plan. They are as follow:

- The First principle is to maintain adequate levels of energy, nutrients, movement, and rest for optimal health
- The Second principle is balancing different food groups, and consuming foods in the right proportion
- The Third principle is consuming the appropriate number of calorie to maintain a healthy weight, depending on your metabolism and exercise levels
- The Fourth principle is focusing on creating a nutrient-dense diet which is less in calories
- The Fifth principle is learning to be moderate with foods which have high fat and sugar content
- The Sixth principle is opting for varieties in your diet besides being rich in nutrients necessary for your health.

Most people relate diets to short-term weight loss and restrictive food intake. However, a diet plan is tailored to an individual's health status, weight and lifestyle, along with their weight loss and health goals.

Nutrition is the process of absorbing macronutrients and micronutrients from foods so that they can help the body grow while keeping it healthy. Healthy or "balanced" nutrition begins by choosing foods from all of the food groups, which includes proteins, carbohydrates, fats, vitamins and minerals. A more varied diet helps the body to meet all of its nutrient needs. Hence diet planning is essential if you are focusing on a healthy and disease-free lifestyle.

Few steps that are essential to plan any diet are as follows:

• **Step-1: Goal Setting**

Setting a goal is very important, be it your carrier choices or your health. Your goal will be the first step in your diet planning process. There are various kinds of goals that people set related to their health. I'll discuss the four commonly set goals; they are as follows:

- ❖ Losing fat
- ❖ Building muscle
- ❖ Overall health with more energy and better digestion
- ❖ Helping with ailments such as type-2 diabetes or clinical diabetes etc

The diet is entirely different for all the four options above. When losing fat as I discussed earlier, you have to consume 10-30 % calories less than your TDEE and 10-15% more than your TDEE while gaining muscle or weight. And when it comes to maintaining your weight, you have to consume calories approximately equal to your TDEE.

If you are going through any medical ailments, first of all, you should take your doctor's advice, whether it is safe for you to lose weight or gain muscle. Then look for the foods you need to avoid in a particular disease. After that, check the value of your TDEE and plan it according to your goal. But it is necessary again to mention that you should always cross-check the diet with your doctor. While planning your diet, you should always monitor your nutritional requirements and your macronutrients intake.

Here is a tip; always paste a written statement of your goals on your fridge or study table or any other places where you can see it many times in a day. It will help you to remember your goals and stop you from cheat diet.

- **Step-2: The Approach**

When I was on my weight loss journey, during the first two months, I avoided all the outside food. I was on a strict diet as I had to get away with my stuck pregnancy weight. But two months later, I started having my favorite foods twice a week as I lost a good amount in initial two months. When I reached my target, I kept my diets very relaxed along with monitoring and tracking my food choices.

So everyone has a different approach to their fitness journey. Approach here means the way you want to keep your weight loss or muscle gain journey. The approach is essential if you are looking for good results. There are various approaches like enjoyable approach, realistic approach and aggressive approach. So choose the method according to your comfort.

Remember it is not necessary to go on a strict diet to lose weight because 95% dieters who lose weight on such a diet tend to gain the weight back, and most of them gain back more than they had initially. You can lose those extra kgs by eating your favorite foods as well. For example, when I was on my weight loss journey, I didn't give up on my food habits; instead, I modified them a little bit and the results were terrific.

So choose the approach that you can keep more extended and suits your lifestyle. It is necessary to learn the differences between these approaches. They are as follow:

1. *Enjoyable Approach*

In this approach, as the word enjoyable suggests, you will have a relaxed diet schedule and thus taking care of your cravings. Many of my clients that opted for this approach don't feel as if they are on a diet. This approach aims at consuming 30% calories of your TDEE which comes from your favorite foods and 70% from healthy foods. Favorite foods can be your junk food like pizzas, burgers, ice creams, alcohol, etc. There are two ways to proceed with this.

Firstly for example; if your TDEE is 2000 calories per day, every day you are having 600 calories from your favorite foods and rest 1400 calories from healthy eating.

While in the second way, what you can do is choose two days a week. And in those two days, you can have your favorite foods while the remaining five days is for healthy eating. So in this way, you get to eat whatever you want and also you won't have to give up on your cravings and hunger. Hence, it is possible to lose weight while eating your favorite foods.

This approach is ideal for people who party a lot or spend their weekends usually eating outside. So yes, here is an eye-opener, if you are a party person or a lover of food, you can still lose weight without giving up totally on your favorite foods.

2. *Realistic Approach*

This approach is the most followed and it gives outstanding results. One of my friends, Shruti, was 10kgs overweight wanted to have one meal of her choice in a week during her weight loss journey. So she followed this approach, and she lost 10kgs in 2.5 months.

The realistic approach is very flexible as in this approach, 20% calories of your TDEE comes from your favorite foods while the rest of the 80% calories will be from healthy foods.

For example; if my TDEE is 2000 and I follow this approach, then 400 calories of my TDEE comes from my favorite foods and rest 1600 calories from healthy food. Again the favorite foods don't mean only the junk foods; instead, it can be either junk or healthy, totally depends on your food choices.

This approach is opted by those who want to keep their meals neither strict nor relaxed, but rather keeping it realistic. This approach is the best; when it comes to giving results as by following this approach, you can sustain with the longer-term consequence.

3. *Aggressive Approach*

As the name suggests, this approach is aggressive and more towards a strict diet. It aims at keeping 10% calories of your TDEE from your favorite foods and rest 90% calories of your TDEE from healthy foods. For example, if my TDEE is 2000 calories, then 200 calories of my TDEE will be from my favorite foods and rest 1800 calories of my TDEE will be from healthy foods.

This approach gives speedy results and mostly preferred by those who aim for tremendous transformation. You get the results very soon in this approach. But to satisfy your hunger and cravings, you get only 200 calories, and that's the pain you have to take if you want fast results.

For example; one of my client lost 7kgs by following this approach in the first two weeks but due to its restricted nature, he later on shifted to the realistic approach.

So in short, you can't predict the approach that will yield good results; it depends on individuals. So choose wisely as the enjoyable process might look slow in giving results, but in the long term, it can give you tangible results.

However, in this aggressive process, you might lose more weight in a short time but the chances are later, you start eating more and again gain weight.

- ## Step-3: Decide the Calorie Target Based on Your Goal

Before starting any diet, it is essential to know about your calorie targets. First of all, you should know what your TDEE is. For this, I told you the easiest way is to use online calculators rather than using lengthy formulas.

After knowing your TDEE, the next thing is to decide your calorie intake depending on your goal; whether you want to lose fat, build muscle or maintain your weight and so on.

For example; if my TDEE is 2000 and I have to lose fat, then my calorie intake should be (10-30) % < TDEE, i.e. I should be consuming between 1400-1800 calories in a day. If I am opting for weight gain or muscle gain diet, then my calorie intake should be (10-15) % > TDEE, i.e. 2200 - 2300 calories per day. And lastly, if I have to maintain my current weight, then I should consume slightly less than or equal to my TDEE, i.e. 2000 calories per day. So this is how you decide your daily calorie intake.

- ## Step-4: Decide Macrosplit And Meal Framework

We all have studied about macronutrients in our school days but very few of us remember the role they play in keeping our body healthy. Your gym instructor must have told you to alter the intake of proteins or cutting carbs or fats for your various goals. But hardly few of us know how much of these nutrients our bodies require.

What are macronutrients?

Macronutrients refer to carbohydrates, fats and protein — the three essential components of every diet. It is crucial to have the right balance of macronutrients in our diet to adhere to healthy diets.

Diets which lack macronutrients or which are high in one macronutrient or less in other, generally are not for everyone. To increase your results on a reduced-calorie diet, it becomes essential to individualize your macronutrient ratio depending on your health and your preferences.

The main reason behind the failure of any diet is that people can't stick with them for long periods.

Therefore, it's essential to follow a reduced-calorie diet that fits your preferences, lifestyle and goals.

The Acceptable Macronutrient Distribution Ranges (AMDR) are:

> Carbohydrates; they constitute 45–65% of your daily calories
> Fats; they constitute 20–35% of your daily caloric intake.
> Proteins; they constitute 10–35% of your daily caloric intake.

How to alter them according to our goals

- **Build muscles**; you should have a diet rich in carbs. For example, you should consume 25% calories from proteins, 25%calories from fats and 50% calories from carbohydrates in your diet.
- **Fat loss;** you should have a diet rich in proteins. For example, you should consume 40% protein, 30% fat, and 30% carbohydrates in your diet.
- **Weight management**; the best macro split is 32% protein, 40% fat, 28% carbohydrates.

In short, you should daily be eating:

> ➢ 2 grams protein per kilo of bodyweight,
> ➢ 0.7 grams – 1.2 grams fats per kilo of bodyweight, and
> ➢ The remaining ones from carbohydrates

If we talk about measuring your macronutrients, then remember this:

1 gram of protein = 4 calories

1 gram of carbohydrate = 4 calories

1 gram of fat = 9 calories

So if you take 100gm of chicken, that doesn't mean it has 100gm of protein. You need to check the labels on food or search on Google. For example; 100gm of chicken has 23gms of protein, 1gm fats, 0gms carbs, so that amounts to (23*4)+(1*9)+(0*4)= 107 calories. So that's what you see within the food.

I have included the macro-splits and the calorie value of different food items we take on a usual basis in the next chapter.

- ## **Step-5: Deciding the Meal Ingredients and Meal Combos**

It is imperative to design the meal ingredients, like the type of foods to select; which food to avoid, which seasonal foods are the best swaps of the expensive off-season foods, what can be readily available and so on. What you need to do is make a list of all core food ingredients you are going to eat and ensure they all are stocked up. While designing a meal, always remember to choose three to six meals and meal combos based on your lifestyle, preferences and availability.

One of my favorite tactics is to use leftover foods to make something healthier and delicious the next day. For instance; whenever I cook dal and brown rice for dinner, it often exceeds the quantity by a little amount while cooking, and it must have happened with you also.

I have seen many people throwing leftovers in the dustbin, which looks awful. My mother always made sure we didn't waste any bite of our food and thanks to her, I am very good at dealing with leftovers. I used it to make either daal parantha or daal kachori for breakfast.

With leftover veggies, I always make a Frankie or a club sandwich. And believe me; your life becomes really easy as you need not start from scratch to prepare a meal. Don't ever disregard leftovers as part of your meal plan strategy. Using the same ingredients for multiple meals doesn't mean they all have to taste the same. This tactic will help to keep your grocery list a little bit shorter, and maybe even help you in lowering your weekly budget.

For examples;

- ❖ If you are buying oats, then you can make many dishes out of one ingredient like oats porridge, oats uttapam, vegetable oats, oats smoothie, oats chilla and many more.

- ❖ We usually have cooked daal for lunch or dinner, but you can make stuffed dal parantha next day as breakfast using leftover dal.

- ❖ When it comes to rice, cooked leftover rice can be turned into yummy idlis or rice parantha next day for breakfast.

- ❖ Similarly, leftover veggies can turn into a vegetable sandwich or nuggets as breakfast or snacks.

So the purpose is to say no to food wastages.

- **Step-6: Cook Your Meals**

Home-cooked food is always better when you are aiming at weight loss. It is also essential that you cook your meals at home as it will not only give you control on all the ingredients such as salt, sugar and oil, but it will help you in counting your calories which is very important while you are aiming for weight loss or muscle gain.

By cooking your meals yourself, you will be cooking in a limited amount because nobody knows better than you that how much you have to eat and this ultimately save the food from wastage and also helps you in portion control of your foods.

Cooking your meals gives you the option of healthy swaps like replacing your sour cream with yoghurt, refined oil with ghee/coconut oil or olive oil and so on. For example; I have a cook at home and I do ask him to do all the chopping, but I always prefer to cook myself according to my way.

Let me tell you a hack; the process of making food diminishes the actual eating experience, which is due to constant smelling and tasting of food. It makes you eat lesser, further helping you to consume more calories, resulting in weight loss. By cooking yourself, you can ensure that you and your family eat fresh and wholesome meals. It will help you to look and feel healthier, boost your energy, stabilize your weight and mood, and improve your sleep and resilience to stress. So it is always recommended to cook your meals yourself unless and until you have a shortage of time.

- ## Step-7: Monitor and Track

One thing I always follow is monitoring my food choices, tracking my food calories and making sure that I am eating the right food in the right quantity. Monitoring and tracking have made my weight loss journey very smooth. Monitoring and tracking are crucial when you are following any diet.

- ❖ First of all, weigh every day. I know most people tell you not to measure your weight every day but believe me, it works. When you measure your weight every day, you remain more conscious about your targets, and this helps in reaching your goal sooner. Weight should be calculated at the same time every day. Weight before and after a workout may differ by 1kgbecause of water loss after the exercise.

❖ Create a progress photograph or take pictures on your phone in your journey and keep them on your wallpaper so that you can remain motivated. I prefer a mirror, as it is the best guide to track your transformation.

❖ Keep tracks of your monthly measurements, i.e. your chest, waist and hip, because sometimes we lose the inches first and then the weight, so vitals are significant.

❖ Keep track of the calories you burn every day. These days, there are so many mobile applications for this, and also fitness bands are available in markets.

❖ Keep track of your calorie intake; the food you eat and a portion of food you consume daily. It is essential to have the calorie count and to keep it in its limit to achieve your goals sooner.

❖ And last but not least, always keep healthy food as your first choice because healthy food will result in good health.

So these seven steps are essential for planning your diet, and one has to keep it in mind for sure while he or she starts to plan any diet. These steps will help you to plan a diet according to your body's nutritional requirements and also keeping the macro-splits in mind. So I hope you had a better understanding of how these few steps will help you plan a diet for yourself, like an expert.

Importance of Macronutrients in Our Bodies

People might have told you to cut on carbs or fats to reduce weight or limit the protein intake, but very few know that these three have their importance in maintaining a healthy body. They shouldn't be ignored; rather, emphasis should be on incorporating them in our diet in the amount which is good for our health.

Why is protein intake important for our body?

Of all the calorie sources, protein has the most significant positive effect on aiding the liver and boosting metabolism. Protein is vital because it maintains muscle mass and bone density. It has the beneficial ability to act in place of glycogen to help burn triglyceride fats.

Protein also contains essential amino acids that further aid the liver in breaking down fat. Since the liver plays a part in so many of the body's vital functions, ailments of the liver are frequently the root cause for many other chronic diseases. So, maintaining a healthy liver isn't just about losing weight; it's about keeping a healthy body overall.

Why are fats essential for our body?

There's a massive misconception that eating fat will make you gain weight. We need essential fats like omega-3swhich our body can't produce on its own. Moreover, fat is vital to our bodies; your body cannot function if it doesn't get high-quality fat.

Fat is also the basis for *myelin* which lines your nerves and allows electricity to flow efficiently in them. You think more quickly when you have more myelin because it allows your nerves to transmit messages faster. Your body also burns fat more efficiently and forms more healthy cell membranes when you consume the right fat.

__Why are carbohydrates essential for our body?__

Carbohydrates are your body's leading source of energy: They act as a fuel for your brain, kidneys, heart muscles, and central nervous system. For instance; fiber is a carbohydrate that aids in digestion, helps you feel full, and keeps blood cholesterol levels in check. Your body can store extra carbohydrates in your muscles and liver for use when you're not getting enough carbohydrates in your diet.

A carbohydrate-deficient diet may cause headache, fatigue, weakness, difficulty in concentration, nausea, constipation, bad breath and vitamin and mineral deficiencies.

In the next chapter, we will be discussing how to count calories in our meals, which will further help you to plan a perfect meal.

Chapter Seven - STEP IV (Monitoring the Calorie Intake)

I remember one of my clients, after taking diets for three consecutive months decided to take a break as he was on his business trip. He lost 12kgs and was super happy with his new body. His food habits were changed, and he was walking 10,000 steps every day. At the end of the third month, he asked how he can maintain the weight, and I told him to be cautious about his calorie intakes. Now the question arises; how to do that?

In this chapter, I'll be telling you how to measure the calories in your foods and also the macronutrients present in them. Tracking your food calories is essential when it comes to maintaining your weight; this person who has lost 12kgs has been maintaining his weight since then just by tracking his calories and eating appropriately.

The diet is planned according to TDEE, i.e. Total Daily Energy Expenditure. But while preparing our meals how will we know the amount of calories the particular food or ingredients contains?

By the end of this chapter, you will be able to understand the amount of calorie you are consuming and whether that consumption is sufficient or satisfying for your nutritional requirements. As I already discussed how much of macro-splits we should consume in a day, keeping its track is essential so that our body remains healthy, nutrients sufficient and disease-free. So now we will discuss how we should deal with the measurements when it comes to foods.

How Do You Measure Your Food?

When you eat your meals, one crucial thing is how much you should consume. I have seen people cooking food, keeping it in the pan and when they are serving, they eat till the entire food until it's finished, but if some amount is left by chance, then thanks to our mother, friend, wife or whosoever is serving; forcefully serving it to you.

That's how we have been doing with our eating habits. After eating so much food, you feel so full and lazy that you rush to hit the bed and sleep. It is not a problem but a big injustice that you might be doing to your health. In this process, you are unknowingly committing three mistakes:

1. You are cooking your food without measuring your ingredients.

2. You are eating more than your hunger so that the food doesn't get wasted, but adding unnecessary calories and fats to your body.

3. And when you are full and feeling heavy, you went to sleep immediately, thus giving an opportunity to those extra calories to turn into accumulating fats in your body.

So to avoid all these mistakes, what I recommend is to always measure your food.

Now there are different ways to do that; some people cook the food and measure with some bowl or cup before eating; this is also known as portion control. Others measure the ingredients before cooking. Well, both the ways are right; it's your choice on how you have to do it.

For example, a friend of mine in Delhi keeps a food weighing machine and supposed that if he planned to eat omelette for breakfast and he had kept 400-500 calories for it, then 50gms of egg means one medium egg.

50gm eggs=1 egg=70cal in which

Protein = 6gms, 1gm protein=4cal and hence 6*4= 24cal from protein

Fats=5gms, 1gm fats= 9cal and hence 5*9= 45cal from fats

Carbs = 0

Total calories= 45+24=69calories in 1 medium egg or 50gms egg

If he took three eggs then, 69* 3=207 calories

For making an omelette, he'll need some oil. So if he uses 10gms of oil which is purely fat and 1gm of fat= 9cal, total cal in 10gm of oil=10*9=90 calories

If he takes two bread toast, then it amounts to 130 calories, in which protein is 3gms, fats are 2gms and carbs are 25gms.

So now his breakfast includes = 207 calories from eggs+ 90 calories from oil+ 130 calories from bread toast= 427 calories.

So that's how you can calculate calories in your food by measuring ingredients.

By this method, you can eat your food by grams, looking at the ingredients, calories and then cooking and consuming it.

There are certain foods that we all consume on an everyday basis which I am attaching in a chart along with their calories and macro-splits measurements. But you cannot measure calories by this method every day, so there is an easy and a preferred way which is the Online Food Tracking Applications. This will be discussed in the next section.

Food Calorie Sheet with Macronutrients Split

Food Items	Quantity	Carbohydrates	Protein	Fats	Calories
Whole Eggs	1 Medium(50 GMS)	0	6	5	69
Cow's Milk	1 Cup (250ML)	11.5	8.3	4	11.5
Almond Milk	1 Cup (250ML)	2	2	4	52
Coconut Milk	1 Cup (250ML)	2	1	4	48
Plain Yoghurt	1 Cup (250ML)	16	12	4	148
Cottage Cheese	1 Cup (250ML)	6	31	11	247

Red Beans(Rajma)	250GMS	40	13	1	221 (COOKED)
Chickpeas (Chole)	250GMS	40	13	1	221 (COOKED)
3Lentils(Dal- All types)	250GMS	37	17	1	225 (COOKED)
Chicken Breast	100GMS	0	30	0	120
Oatmeal	50GMS	38	8	3	191
Fish Of Choice	100GMS	0	21	3	111
Tuna (Canned)	100GMS	0	26	0	104
Quinoa	50GMS	34	7	2	182
Whole Wheat Bread	2 Medium Slices	25	3	2	130
Potatoes	100GMS	20	1.8	2	105
Brown Rice	100GMS	22	3	2	118
Chapatti	1 Medium	20	3	1	101
Whole Wheat Pasta	50 GMS	37	7	1	185
Apple	1 Medium	20	0	0	80
Banana	1Medium	9	2	15	160
Honey	1 Tablespoon	10	0	0	40
Peanut Butter	1Tablespoon	2	3	7	80
Desi Ghee	1 Tablespoon	0	0	15	135

Extra-Virgin Olive Oil	1 Tablespoon	0	0	15	135
Almonds	1oz	5	6	14	170
Walnuts	1oz	3	4.5	18	192
Flaxseeds	1 Tablespoon	10	7	10	158
Dates	1	6	0.2	0.3	28
Extra-Virgin Coconut Oil	1 Tablespoon	0	0	15	135

This list of ingredients will help you to measure the calories and nutrients in your meals on a daily basis.

Using Mobile Applications to Measure Your Food Calories

Another method to measure your food calories is using mobile applications. It is the easiest and the most preferred method as by this, you save your precious time.

Various applications like HealthifyMe, Cron-o-meter, MyFitnessPal etc. are available these days to serve the purpose. These apps help you to track your food, exercises, weight/waist progress, water consumption and macros. Whether you want to lose weight, tone up, get healthy or change your habits, these apps help you to track your overall food intake, your calories and also track your water intake.

Keeping yourself hydrated is the first and foremost step in losing weight as it helps to flush out all the toxins. So these apps also remind you to have a glass of water at specific intervals to complete your target of 3ltrs per day.

So now we know how to measure the calorie intakes from foods and macro-splits so that we can keep a watch on our meals and eat according to our TDEE, and the goals we want to achieve while keeping in mind the body's nutritional requirements intact.

In the next chapter, I will be giving you sample diet plans.

Chapter Eight - STEP V (Sample Diet Plan)

When it comes to meal planning, I always plan a weekly schedule and then according to the results of previous weeks, I design the next week's plan. So basically, a month plan includes four diet plans.

Here, I will be sharing a one-week sample diet plan according to different goals, so these diet plans can act as a starting point of your diet planning journey. This can also be taken as a reference point through which you can design your next meal plans.

Planning a diet is easy as you just have to calculate your TDEE and decide your goals and plan accordingly. Certain principles need to be followed for this diet plan such as:

- If you have any disease or ailment, you can always cross-check with your doctor.

- If you have any food allergies, then just swap that food with another having the same nutrient value.

- It is not mandatory to follow only these foods; I have just given you a basic idea on how a meal plan works. I have mentioned just a sample diet so that you have a basic idea of how the diet is planned. So depending on your activity level, your TDEE and your goals, you can modify it.

WEEK-1: WEIGHT LOSS PLAN

Sandhya is 35 years of age and has a very sedentary lifestyle. She is 150cms in height and weighs around 68kgs. She wants to lose 18kgs of weight. Her TDEE is 1556 calories per day.

Since we know that for weight loss, one should consume (10-30%) < TDEE, she needs to consume between 1100 calories to 1400 calories depending on her approach.

Let's frame a meal plan for her.

On Waking Up	1 Glass of Cumin and Coriander seeds water (7cal) + 1 Glass of lukewarm water 5 Almonds and 1 Walnut (soaked) (68cal)
Breakfast	2 Eggs Omelette or in any form (207cal) with two slices of brown bread (148cal) **Or** One bowl of Black chana chaat with lots of cucumber, onion, tomato and lemon with a pinch of rock salt (210cal) + 2 bread toast (148)
Mid Morning	2 Oranges **Or** Two sweet lime (Mosambi) (126cal)
Lunch	30mins before lunch: 1 cucumber + 1 tomato+ some radish salad (15cal) MEAL: 1-2 Multigrain flour

	chapattis (2 chapatti = 165cal) with one bowl of any green vegetable (140cal) 30mins post-lunch: 1 Glass of cumin and coriander seeds water(7cal)
Mid Evening	Green Tea + a handful of roasted fox nuts (55.5cal) or one apple (86cal)
Dinner	Pre dinner: 1 cucumber and some radish salad (15 calories) Meal: 1 Multigrain bread club sandwich (190cal) **Or** One bowl of Vegetable Buckwheat (186.6cal) Bed Time: 1 Glass of lukewarm lemon water with one crushed Garlic Turi (3cal)

So if you add the total calories, it will come around 1150 calories in a day.

WEEK-1: WEIGHT GAIN PLAN

Tanishka is 25 years old and is 5 feet and 8 inches. She weighs around 55kgs. She is getting married in a few months and has to gain some weight. Her lifestyle is very active and her TDEE is 1800 calories per day.

So for weight gain, she needs to consume (10-30%) > TDEE. That mean she should have between 1900 to 2400 calories per day.

On Waking Up	10 soaked Almonds with the peels (78cal)
Breakfast	Banana Almond smoothie (316cal) + 1 bowl of vegetable daliya (83cal) / vegetable oats (88cal)
Mid Morning	Any 2 fruits (100-150cal) + 1 glass of lassi (198cal)

Lunch	2 chapattis (2 chapatti has 170 cal) / 1 bowl of rice (180 cal) + vegetables (120cal) + dal/paneer/egg (130cal) + 1 small bowl of curd (90cal)
Mid Evening	1 glass of Banana milkshake (230cal) + bhelpuri/upma/grilled sandwich (202cal)
Dinner	Pre dinner: vegetable soup/chicken soup (60cal) Meal: 2 chapattis (170cal) + vegetables (120cal) + 1 small bowl of dal/non-veg (chicken/egg/fish) (130cal) + 1 small bowl of curd (90cal) Bed time: 1 glass of golden milk(120cal)

So this meal plan amounts to around 2300 calories per day.

These two are sample 1 week diet plan designed for weight loss and weight gain. These diet plans are designed to take in mind the food choices and lifestyle of the concerned client. These will give you a clear picture on how to create meal plans. So plan your meals and get your fitness journey started by none other than you. While following your diets, don't forget to keep yourself hydrated.

In the next chapter, we will discuss some food hacks that will make your diets enjoyable.

PART III - Making Your Journey Enjoyable

Chapter Nine - Food Hacks

I remember sitting in a coffee shop with my friend. While recollecting the old memories, we ordered our coffee. She is now settled in Bombay and was in Delhi for her project work. Let me tell you, she is a chatterbox. She can talk about Vada Pav, Bhel Puri, Aaloo Tikki for hours nonstop.

After all her foodie talks, she asked me how I plan a diet, and without waiting for my answer, she instantly said, "I can't diet even a single day, I can't give up on my taste buds, hunger and cravings". I laughed and asked "who told you that diet means giving up on hunger and cravings".

I told her that, "the diet plan doesn't mean I have to keep my clients starving or don't give importance to their craving". She replied that "diet food is like eating salads green leafy vegetables sprouts and boiled food". And I was shocked to hear this. I was about to explain to her but suddenly, a waiter came and served us our coffees, I offered her a sip from my coffee. She tasted and said, "Wow it's so yummy". I took a deep breath because along with it; she got all her answers.

She asked me which one I ordered, and I replied her that it's the same with what I used to have but with a slight change. I just asked them to make my coffee in almond milk instead of regular milk. I told her that "we both are having coffees, but you are consuming 300 calories, and I have just 140 calories with a better taste".

And that's what I do in diets; I just follow some food hacks and some healthy swaps and present it in the form of a meal plan to my clients to satisfy their, hunger, cravings, and they get most of the nutrients.

Most of us think the same way about diets. So my chatterbox friend turned into a patient listener and admitted that being a foodie doesn't mean you have to consume unhealthy foods. She asked me if she can also reduce some weight, and I told her "why not?" When a mother of eight months can do it effortlessly then why can't you? I gave her some food hacks and made her aware of the healthy swaps she can follow in her daily diets and can get magic results from it.

What are food hacks?

One day, my husband told me that "few friends are coming for dinner tonight, so we will order from a good restaurant" as they have Punjabi taste buds so "kuch tadakta bhadakta chalega." And he was also worried as he is so health-conscious that he doesn't want to cheat diet, so I ensured him not to worry. I asked him not to order from the restaurant, and I decided to organize a homemade dinner.

This pandemic has made me more skeptical about hygiene in the restaurants. I asked him not to worry and leave the food portion to me. I asked him to prepare a list of songs for karaoke so that we can have a fun singing night. I knew there would be kids, so pizza and pasta are everyone's favorite, and "tadakta bhadkta" as my husband mentioned, reminded me of dal makhani, shahi paneer, naan.

Yeah, you are reading right, this is a nutritionist talking. Now see the swaps and hacks I followed:

- Daal makhani was made with homemade white butter instead of cream and oil

- Shahi paneer was replaced with tofu in palak curry with homemade butter and ghee instead of refined oil and cream and still more shahi

- Refined flour naan was replaced with ragi jowar and pudina chapatti

- The typical pizza was replaced with rice flour base pizzas

- The pasta was replaced with Zucchini noodles

So this was our healthy dinner menu which was more nutritious. You won't believe how these minor changes not only made us eat healthily but also tastier, and I still remember how everyone felt; mesmerized by dinner.

So there are some more food hacks which I follow in my daily routine and would like to share them with you. First of all, say a strict NO to the following foods:

* **Refined sugar** - the worst thing ever
* **Refined flour**- just remove it from your kitchen
* **Sugar sweetened beverages**- unhealthiest foods on the planet
* **White bread** - highly refined with a lot of sugar added, results in weight gain and obesity
* **Candy bars**-extremely unhealthy, pack a lot of added sugar, refined oils, refined flour
* **Fruit juices**- loaded with sugar and highly processed
* **Ice cream**- avoid eating it in massive amounts

I swap refined sugar with honey or jaggery. I even love beat my coffee in jaggery whenever I want to add sweetness to my coffee. I always try to use multigrain flour or jowar, ragi and bajra instead of the wheat flour. Let me mention that these millets are incredible for our health besides being cheaper.

Whenever it comes to sugar-sweetened beverages, I always prefer to have whole fruits rather than juices, thus staying away from processed drinks. White bread is a big NO in my house; instead, I prefer to have multigrain or whole-grain bread. When it comes to candy bars, I always prefer dark chocolate with little or no sweetness to satisfy my taste buds.

Here are some hacks.

• Hack 1 - False hunger alarm

Have you ever felt hungry after 1-1.5 hrs of having your meals? I usually feel this and couldn't wait to rush to the refrigerator to grab what I can have. This must-have happened to you because I used to go through this feeling every day. But wait, I had a proper meal, I was full also, then why I am feeling hungry so soon?

And after eating unnecessary food, you might feel guilty. Yes! And what if I say you don't need to have food at that time? Let me tell you a hack. When this happened with me for 3-4 days, I followed a hack; instead of having food; I had plenty of water and guess what? After that, I didn't felt like having anything.

I want you to follow this hack, and if after having a glass of water your hunger vanishes, then consider that it was nothing but your body reminding you to have water by giving you a false hunger alarm.

- ## **Hack 2 - Choosing brown rice over white rice**

I remember before being a nutritionist, I used to consume wheat flour, white rice, white bread and many such refined things. Whenever I heard of people eating brown rice or multigrain flour, I used to think "are these mad or what?" I mean "brown rice mai vo taste kaha jo white rice mai hai". And I know many of you feel the same way.

Some people consider brown rice to be less in calories, that's why whenever they choose to diet, the first thing they do is to shift from white to brown rice. But if that's the reason for switching your rice with brown rice, then you are conceptually wrong. Let me tell you that why I always prefer brown rice over white rice:

White rice	**Brown rice**
• Processed	• Whole grain
• Enriched with vitamins and minerals	• Naturally contains vitamins and minerals
• High glycemic index	• Low glycemic index
• Less fiber	• More fiber

Though the caloric difference is minor between the two when it comes to health benefits, brown rice proves better than white rice; being a whole grain with bran and germ attached to it unlike refined white rice and more fibrous, makes it helpful to lower cholesterol, helps in moving waste through the digestive tract, promotes fullness, and may help in preventing the formation of blood clots.

So if you feel convinced with this, give it a try, and I am sure you will fall in love with brown rice like I do.

• HACK 3 - Cooking in less oil makes the food tastier

During my childhood when my mother used to cook food for us, I, like most of the kids was always curious to know what ingredients are going into the kadhai and cooker as those colorful ingredients were always pleasing to eyes. I used to ask one question every time; "why we add oil in meals", and she used to reply that she does so to make it tastier.

And this is the belief of every household; that to make food more delicious, add more refined oil. These days, various brands are also coming up with the idea of introducing heart-healthy oil. But I wonder; can refined oil be heart healthy?

The answer is NO. Instead, replace your refined oil with extra virgin olive oil or coconut oil or ghee. Cooking can be done in 1tsp also rather than 2-3tbsp. You won't believe food will be tastier with less oil.

• HACK 4 - Desi ghee help you lose weight

As a child, I used to wait for my summer vacations to begin so that I could go to my nana- Nani's place, and I know every kid grows up with this feeling. But my excitement was a bit different, let me tell you how.

My maternal grandparents were having two cows and one calf which they kept for themselves. So my Nana always wanted us to have organic milk and ghee. But as we grew up, especially we girls, became so conscious about losing weight and maintaining our shape that the first thing that we avoid eating was, ghee. And my Nani used to scold me so much for this by saying "ghee haddiyo ke liye bhautr jariuri hai". And I think many of you must have heard the same dialogue. And yes it's so true, although I realized it a bit later. Many of us while dieting believes ghee will make us fat, but ironically it helps in losing fat, lowers blood pressure and improves gut health. So ghee is essential for you.

While on my weight loss journey, I always made sure that I am having 1tsp of ghee regularly in my diet and I managed to lose 20kgs. You can either cook it with your meals, or you can just add it to the top of your dal or sabzi.

- ### **HACK 5 - The magical oats**

In the past few months, one significant change I have done in my life is replacing corn flakes or chocos with oats. Isn't it boring? Yes, many of you might think the same way.

One of my clients, Arushi, completed her 1st-week plan and texted me her vitals so that I can give her the next week plan. So when I sent her the plan, I asked if there's anything she wanted to change. And without giving it a thought, she said oats as she didn't like the taste. I could have easily changed it, but I want my clients not to give up easily. I asked her how she prepares oats, and she replied "ismei prepare ka kuch hai bhi, boiled milk mai daalo aur khalo". And that was when I wondered how badly we are treating this fantastic food. I know you must have been doing the same thing, but don't worry.

So I told her that whenever I have to eat oats, I experiment with it like making oatmeal loaded with fruits, the yummiest oats uttapam, oats upma, oats veggie bowl, oats spinach chilla. She was amazed when she heard this and asked me not to change the food, and that week she tried many recipes. And to this day, she waits for the plan which contains oats. So I want you to experiment with food. As far as oats are concerned, I swapped this with other items because of its rich antioxidant properties. It is highly nutritious, lowers cholesterol levels, controls blood sugar and aids in weight loss.

- ## **HACK 6 - Jaggery over refined sugar**

Many of you who have a sweet tooth might think that if we are on a diet, we will have to give up on sweets. My husband like many of us used to fear a lot about following a diet plan as he is so fond of sweets that I have to keep something like ladoo or halwa in my kitchen so that he can have some after lunch or dinner.

I am not in favor of having refined sugars which these sweets contain, so it always worried me. When he decided to go on a weight loss journey, what I did was replaced white sugar with jaggery which has more antioxidants, his sweets intake was diverted to a cube of dark chocolate or 1-2 dates per day.

Believe me; now, he was more happy and contented as this sweetness was doing benefits for his health rather than deteriorating it. You will thank yourself your entire life for these great swaps as they aid in weight loss also. Even if you want to have Indian sweets, opt for ladoo made of multigrain flours, nuts, ghee and jaggery.

- ## **HACK 7 - The twisty salad**

I remember one of my clients, Nimisha on receiving her diet plan said salads are boring, and eating them before meals are tough. She was not fond of salads, then I asked her how she always prepared her salads, and the answer she gave was so expected and common.

So what we do is cut the round slices of cucumber tomato, radish or carrot and put them separately in the plate rather than mixing as if they all are annoyed from each other, and now we expect ourselves to finish it. Even I can't finish it that way.

Always remember, if you make food pleasing to your eyes, you will be able to finish it soon. So let me tell you a hack to deal with this situation. When it comes to salad, I chop tomato-cucumber, lettuce, carrot, and broccoli in small pieces and mix them all. Then I will squeeze half a lemon in it, add some herbs, chili flakes, oregano, and some pink salt and mix it well.

You can also add mustard sauce if you have and sometimes diet mayonnaise to enrich the flavors. By doing so, I promise you; your salad bowl will never remain unfinished. I always eat my salad 30 minutes prior to the meal and this is the routine I never break.

Eating salads before a meal helps to increase vegetable intake, and also increases our fiber intake which helps to reduce our bad cholesterol. And if you are aiming at weight loss or healthy weight management, then adequate intake of fiber is essential. It also normalizes bowel movements and even controls blood sugar levels.

- ## **HACK 8 - Snacks don't mean pakoda/fritters only**

One day, I invited my friend Shruti for tea. So I asked her "what snacks will you prefer with your evening tea"? She said "anything yaar, bhujiya-biscuits chal jaenge". When I insisted, she said it's about to rain "pakode bana lete hai".

So I prepared pakodas for her and some roasted fox-nut chaat, some corns and bhuna chana dipping with pita bread. When she came home, I served her the evening tea with snacks. She said, "kya kha rahi hai pakode khaa aur maje le". And I offered her fox-nut chaat and pita bread with dipping, and she liked it so much that she left the pakodas and ate what I made for myself.

She asked for the recipe then and there as she couldn't believe how easy and healthy snacks can be so tasty besides providing so many health benefits.

Yes, this is the problem with everyone; we presume that diet food do not taste good, but I want you to try at least because there are so many experiments you can do with just basic things.

I always recommend roasted fox-nuts, bhuna chana, corn chaat, avocado egg salad, peanut butter banana bites and many more to my clients for their evening snacks and they are so happy with it. But you have to start somewhere to get the health benefits.

• HACK 9 - Healthy cookies

Before starting my weight loss journey, I remember I couldn't give up on chocolate cookies. Chocolate cookies and cakes were an all-time favorite. I remember my husband saying that "how will you manage without these cookies?" and I replied, "Let's see, I will try not to have it".

It happens with many of us, trying to give up on our cravings for losing weight. But what if I say we have an equally tasty alternative? Let me share my experience with you.

I remember one night; I was craving for a chocolate cookie. I searched the refrigerator and found peanut butter and Marie gold biscuits. I wondered what I was going to do with it so I applied peanut butter on one Marie gold biscuit and kept the other one on top of it, I had a bite and it was so yummy.

From then and there, it has become my cookie swap forever. And after that, I started experimenting on cookies; I tried banana, oatmeal cookies with the natural sweetness of banana, oatmeal dark choco-chip cookies and many more. The idea is not to use refined flour, refined oil and refined sugar while preparing cooking.

• HACK 10 - The healthy pizza

I remember how at midnight, I used to have bad cravings for fast foods during my pregnancy. I have placed an order even at 3am for burgers. It even continued after my delivery. I used to be a big-time lover of burgers and pizza, and I know many of you are. But does dieting means giving up on fast food? No, but it means giving up on refined ingredients. Yes, there are bad for your health; I will say they are the nothing less than slow poison. So how do I fulfill my craving for fast foods?

What I do while making pizzas; I never use refined flour dough. Instead, I prefer rice flour dough or leftover multigrain chapatti and the results are better than the regular pizzas you eat.

Whenever my husband wants to have a burger, I just make Bombay sandwich from wholegrain bread, and I swear it's so yummy that you will forget to eat a burger.

While preparing a sandwich, replace your mayonnaise with mustard sauce. When it comes to noodles, always prefer zucchini noodles or wheat noodles, and same goes for pasta. And always try to keep it as your meal like I have planned for myself that I will have Bombay sandwich or pizza or noodles for dinner and not all of them together. The quantity is significant, so take care of it and do not overeat.

These are some of the hacks that have made my diet life enjoyable, and I do not crave for food because I have found out my healthy swaps. Diets are never dull if you are a little bit smart with food hacks. These hacks have made my life more comfortable, plus they are easy to adapt in your life. There are many food hacks which I follow in my daily routine, but I have listed only the major ones. I hope you adjust them in your food habits and enjoy your diets like my clients and I do.

In the next chapter, I will talk about how to plan your cheat meals because cheat meals are necessary to boost up your mood.

Chapter Ten - How to Plan Your Cheat Meals

While scrolling Instagram, I came across many posts of various actors and actresses regarding cheat meals or binge eating, especially when it's Sunday. Also, whenever I give diet plans to my clients, the one question that bothers everyone is "when can I have a cheat day?"

So yes, when it comes to diets, the most common thought that runs in our minds is regarding the cheat diet. Cheating within a diet should always be on a calculated basis and should be planned just like your diet plan. Some people prefer to have a cheat meal while others go for a cheat day.

What is a cheat meal?

Cheat meal is referred to as a single meal of your food choice that differs from your planned diet. While a cheat day involves free food choices for your entire day.

Cheat diet varies from person to person due to their different taste buds. They are typically high-calorie foods which are generally not allowed in your diet plan. Cheat meal also depends on the diet you follow, like some diets are so strict that they don't allow room for a cheat meal; like the ketogenic diet.

When I started my weight loss journey, my goal was to reduce 15-20kgs and therefore, I was very strict with my diet. So initially, for two months I didn't cheat my diet, but later on I kept one meal in a week as my cheat meal. As I reached my goal, I kept a day in a week as my cheat day. On that day I eat and drink what I want. It is my day where there is no restriction on foods and drinks, and I enjoy the food as a reward to the progress I have made in my weight loss journey without any guilt.

Why should you plan a cheat meal?

We now know that weight loss occurs when you burn more calories than you eat. If you can execute a well-planned diet, then cheat diet is very important for you as a reward.

One of my clients, Sneha was following her diet very strictly for two months, whenever I asked about her food choices, her reply was the same, 'Ma'am you plan whatever is best for me'. She was 8kgs overweight, and after two months she reduced 6.5kgs, and I asked her whether she wanted a cheat day or not, and she said "after achieving my target I'll go for cheat diet".

Then I forcefully requested her to go on one day cheat meal and told her to eat whatever she has been craving for. The reason why I did so was because I noticed that people become bored with the same monotonous schedule. She used to avoid going to parties and get-togethers, and I didn't want anyone to sacrifice their social circle in the process of losing weight. The next day, she texted and said thanks to me and was eager to start her next week's plan.

So your inner happiness matters a lot to achieve your targets. If you are doing good on your weight loss journey, don't take cheat diet as a matter of guilt but rather take it as a reward.

Let me tell you some scientific facts also regarding cheat diet. Some of you might have heard about the hormone leptin, which is responsible for suppressing the feeling of hunger. Whenever we experience significant weight loss, this leptin hormone levels may decrease, due to which we are more likely to overeat with low circulating leptin levels.

It happens because now, you don't have enough hormone levels to send signals to the brain that you are full and satisfied, thus may result in weight gain. So according to various research and studies, it has been said that higher-calorie foods occasionally will trick your hormone cycle and result in producing more leptin temporarily and prevent your desire for overeating.

It is always recommended not to go on a rigorous diet, rather keep one day or one meal in a week for your favorite foods.

How to deal with your cheat diet

While planning your cheat diet, there are some points that you must remember. They are as follows:

- Be smart with your cheat diet. In the initial days, always plan to have a cheat diet once in 2-3 weeks.
- If you want to save yourself from overeating, then prefer eating some nuts or a salad bowl before your cheat meal.

- While choosing a cheat meal, always make sure to opt for the food you wanted to eat for long while or the food you are craving for, to treat you well.
- After a cheat meal, don't punish yourself with extreme physical exercise or guilt. Feel happy, have plenty of water and take a walk for 20-30mins.

I remember when I first had my cheat diet, I couldn't control myself and I ate a lot. The next day I was feeling guilty and uncomfortable that after every meal, I rushed to weighing machine to see how much I have gained.

Well, this might have happened with you also or will happen with you on your first cheat diet. But if you start planning a cheat meal once in 2-3weeks, then you will notice that you are automatically able to control your appetite and will choose the more nutritious foods rather than refined carbohydrates.

So one hack that is there to enjoy your cheat meals that is; plan your cheat days as apart of your diet by fixing it little by little, so it will be easy for you and you will possibly not end up overeating.

Some rules to remember on cheat days

- **Use moderation:** make sure you don't eat like you are eating it for the last time, have 500-1000 calories over your daily intake.
- **Use every 2-3 weeks:** use them only when you feel the need to have a cheat meal; don't compromise with your weight loss progress.
- **Eat veggies and proteins until cheat meal:** this way you will save some calories so you could go carb-crazy.
- **Plan it on a training day:** this way, your body will use some of those extra calories for recovery process from the workout.
- **Do not feel guilty:** don't mess up your cheat meals by getting emotional. Be in the moment and realize that you are rewarding yourself for the goals you achieved.

DETOX DRINKS

My husband went to a party with his colleagues and he ate a lot of fast foods and junk which he didn't plan to eat. Next day on waking up, he felt so heavy and he asked me to help him. I gave him a detox drink and planned his detox day. And by the end of the day, he felt so fresh and light.

Detoxification is a process in which we use some particular foods or drinks that claim to rid your body of toxins, cleansing your digestive tract, improving your health and aids weight loss. Our body is continuously working in clearing out all the unwanted toxins from various organs.

Sometimes we opt for unhealthy food choices like alcohol, caffeine, fast food etc. that are part of modern life which puts unnecessary pressure on our gut and various other organs. It becomes necessary to take out some time and cleanse our body's vital organs from multiple toxins that will help in long term prevention of diseases and thus leaving our body with tremendous energy, better skin and good gut health.

What are the signs that indicate much-needed detox?

- You are unnecessarily stressed, or you feel low on energy even after having good meals

- There are frequently occurring skin problems like pimples, blemishes, breakouts
- You suffer from frequent headaches, or you are on some medication
- Your food choices are unhealthy, like a lot of processed meats, refined carbohydrates, junk food, sweetened beverages, alcohol etc. or you are having problems with digestion
- You have excess body weight, or you are depressed, lacking energy or unmotivated towards your health

If you are facing any of the above problems, then your body needs to have some detoxification and believe me, it works.

There was a time I was suffering from frequent headaches for a week, and I was so disappointed that after trying medication and visiting doctors, I couldn't find a solution. Then I thought of opting for a detox meal plan for 2-3 days and the results were amazing.

Since then, I decided to have detox once in two to three weeks, and now my headaches are gone, and I feel much better than before. Here I am sharing a detox plan, which you can try for 2-3 days and see the results.

Breakfast

- Take 1 cup water
- 1 tbsp flax seeds
- 1 cup raspberries
- One banana
- ¼ cup spinach
- 1 tbsp peanut butter
- 2 tsp lemon juice
- Blend them in a mixer and drink it.

Lunch

- Take ½ cup almond milk
- Four celery stalks
- One cucumber
- 1 cup kale
- ½ green apple
- ½ squeezed lime
- 1 tbsp melted coconut oil
- 1 cup pineapple
- Blend them in a mixer and drink.

Dinner

- Take 1 ½ cups of coconut water
- 1 cup blueberries
- ½ cup mango
- 1 cup kale
- 1tbsp lemon'1/4 avocado
- 1/4tsp cayenne pepper
- 1 tbsp flaxseeds
- Blend them in a mixer and drink.

That's all about the cheat meals and detox drinks. I hope you follow the guidelines and incorporate these simple tips in your schedule. The cheat meals will make your diet plans enjoyable and easy to follow.

In the next chapter, I will introduce some super-foods that one should include in his/her diet to get some excellent health benefits.

Chapter Eleven – Super Foods

Whenever you think of a diet, you want one that is rich in vitamins, minerals, antioxidants so that you can keep your body fit and healthy. When you consume these nutrient-rich foods, they won't only keep you healthy and fit but also keep your body away from some chronic ailments. We have always heard people saying that "include the super foods in your diet to feel great, look good, young and make your body healthy". But what are the super foods? Are they any particular food that is available in supermarkets or big stores? Or is it some kind of supplements?

Instead, these are the super nutritious foods that contain antioxidants and phytochemicals (chemicals responsible for smell and color), vitamins and minerals, most of which are plant-based except fish and dairy.

What are the benefits of including super foods in your diet?

The super foods are rich in vitamins, minerals and having antioxidants which help in keeping your body away from certain diseases and also keeps you fit and healthy. When these foods are included in your balanced diet, they do wonders like helping you with the weight loss. They also keep the heart healthy, thus keeping you away from cardiovascular diseases; promotes healthy brain functions, curbs hunger and cravings, boost up your immune system, prevent diabetes and digestive problems.

Super foods are also known to protect your organs from toxins, help lower cholesterol, regulate metabolism and reduce inflammation. Super foods should always be added to your well-balanced diet. When adding super foods to your diet, be aware that unprocessed, natural varieties offer the most benefits. Foods can quickly lose their nutrient-rich superiority when processed or sugar is added for flavor.

Popular Super foods

There are some popular super foods I'll discuss in this section which are always present around you or are available in your kitchen, but you are not aware of the magical benefits they offer for our health.

- **Turmeric**

Turmeric is also known as the Indian gold and has a history of medicinal use.

Key nutrients: Curcumin and Aromatic-Turmeron

Health benefits of turmeric are many, which include: anti-inflammatory, anti-fungal, anti-oxidant. It has a high potential against various diseases such as diabetes, arthritis, allergies, and Alzheimer. It also helps in increasing neural stem cell growth in the brain by as much as 80%.

Ways to add it in your diet

- ✓ Add it in any curry you consume
- ✓ Add one tablespoon of turmeric powder in milk, boil it and consume.

- **Walnuts**

Also known as the king of nuts and it is said that 1 quarter cup of walnuts provides 100% value of plant-based omega three fatty acids required in a day.

Key nutrients: Plant-based omega 3's ALA (Alpha-linolenic acid), Copper, Manganese, Molybdenum, Biotin, Vitamin-E, Folate.

Health benefits of walnuts: Decreases risk of cardiovascular disease; reduces risk of heart disease due to amino acids present in them, cuts breast cancer risk in half, supports brain health.

Ways to add it in your diet

- ✓ Eat as a snack or soak them I water overnight and have them early morning.
- ✓ You can also sprinkle them on oat meals.

- **Coconut Oil**

It is one of the healthiest foods on the planet.

Key nutrients: Medium Chain Triglycerides (MCT) which contains Caprylic acid, lauric acid, capric acid.

Health benefits of coconut oil: As most of the fats we consume takes longer to digest, this contains MCT which is a perfect source of energy because they only have to go through a 3 step process to be done as fuel rather than other fats which have to go through 26-step process. It boosts immune system, curbs hunger and cravings thus helping with the weight loss. It promotes healthy brain function and results in healthy skin and hair.

Ways to add it in your diet

- ✓ Cook with cold-pressed coconut oil
- ✓ Apply on body, or use for a mouth rinse.

- **Fatty Fishes**

These are also called fabulous fats.

Key Nutrients: Omega-3 contains three types of acids, i.e. ALA (Alpha-linolenic acid) which is plant based, DHA (Docosahexaenoic acid) which is animal-based and Eicosapentaenoic Acid, which is also animal-based.

So, fatty fish are the best sources of the three most crucial omega-3s (EPA and DHA). These fatty acids are considered good fats, unlike the bad saturated fats in meat.

Health benefits: Improves brain function and important for cognitive function, reduces inflammation and reduces risk of chronic diseases.

Ways to add it in your diet

- ✓ Eat a different variety of fish twice a week
- ✓ Else supplement your diet with fish oil or better yet krill oil.

- **Avocados**

This is an excellent food if you're following a low carb diet or keto diet. It is high healthy in fats rather than sugars and is loaded with fiber.

Key nutrients: Vitamin K, Folate, Potassium, Vitamin B5 and Vitamin B6.

Health benefits: they are loaded with oleic acid, which are mono-saturated fatty acids, loaded with fiber which is fantastic for digestion, reduces the risk of heart diseases.

Ways to add it in your diet

- ✓ Can use avocado oil for cooking- stable at high temperature
- ✓ Blend it in smoothies
- ✓ Include it in salads

- **Ghee**

It is a form of clarified butter.

Key nutrients: Conjugated linoleic acid (CLA), Butyric acid, fat-soluble vitamins A, E, K

Health benefits of ghee: Helps in lowering inflammation, blood pressure; improves gut health and digestion; helps in reducing body fat.

Ways to add ghee in your diet

✓ Use it as cooking oil.

- **Blueberries**

Blueberries are always on top when it comes to antioxidant content. Antioxidants are vital for our body as they prevent our body from damage by free radicals.

Key nutrients: Vitamin K, vitamin- C, manganese, anthocyanin flavonoids

Health benefits: lowers blood pressure, helps in fighting cancer, boost brain health, and also prevent ageing due to the presence of berry poly-phenols.

Ways to add it in your diet

- ✓ Blend it in your smoothies
- ✓ Sprinkle it over your oat meals.

- **Matcha Green Tea**

It is a tea which has 15 times more anti-oxidants than blueberries and three times more antioxidants than any A-grade green tea and 137 times more antioxidants than any low-grade Green tea.

Key nutrients: Vitamin K, Vitamin C, Manganese, Anthocyanin flavonoids

Health benefits: helps in lowering your blood pressure, helps in fighting cancer and boosts brain health.

Ways to add it in your diet

- ✓ Blend it in smoothies
- ✓ Sprinkle it over your oatmeal
- ✓ Brew a cup of green tea latte

- **Broccoli**

Broccoli is always on top of my super foods list. It contains several antioxidants that can help in cleaning excessive estrogen, which encourages higher testosterone levels and increases muscle growth.

Key nutrients: Vitamin-K, Vitamin-C, Iron, Fiber, contains a compound called sulforaphane which helps in fighting cancer.

Health benefits: lowers blood pressure, prevents cancer and boost eye health

Ways to add it in your diet

- ✓ Use in salads or you can eat them with other veggies
- ✓ You can add it as an ingredient while making chicken or eggs.

- **Spinach**

Spinach is loaded with antioxidants which help in reducing oxidative stress due to free radicals. Oxidative stress increases the risk of diabetes, cancer and accelerates ageing. Spinach also contains high amounts of ziathene and lutene which are responsible for colors in veggies.

Key nutrients: Vitamin A, Vitamin c, Vitamin k1, fiber, folic acid and calcium

Health benefits: lowers oxidative stress, cancer prevention, boost eye health, lowers blood pressure

Ways to add it in your diet

- ✓ Can be used in salads or cook palak ka saag
- ✓ Some people also use it as an ingredient in chicken and eggs

- **Whole Eggs**

Egg yolk doesn't only raise your cholesterol, it also raises the good cholesterol, i.e. HDL not LDL.

Key Nutrients: Vitamin A, Folate, vitamin b2, vitamin B12, phosphorous, selenium

Health benefits: contains choline which is important to build cell membranes, helps build muscle and lowers body fat.

Ways to add it in your diet

- ✓ Can be enjoyed anytime of the day in the form of Omlette or in boiled form

- **Raw cow milk**

This is in my everyday routine. Yes, a glass of raw cow milk does wonders for your health.

Key nutrients: Vitamin A, Vitamin D, Vitamin K2, CLA, Butyric acid and probiotics

Health benefits: raw cow milk helps with gut's health by optimizing gut bacteria, provides high quality protein for muscle building; supports brain health and nervous system development, helps ease symptoms of colon cancer, IBS, and other intestinal infections.

Ways to add raw cow milk in your diet

- ✓ Prepare oats in it
- ✓ Enjoy by making a protein smoothie.

- **Garlic**

This is one of the ingredients I had been avoiding in my foods for years because of its smell, but as soon as I knew about its health benefits, it is now the first ingredient that never goes off my mind while preparing any meal.

Key nutrients: Vitamin C, Manganese, Vitamin B6, Selenium

Health benefits: lowers blood sugar due to a compound called allicin, reduces cholesterol levels, massively helps with cold and flu, can help prevent Alzheimer's disease and dementia.

Ways to add garlic in your diet

- ✓ You can add them to any of your dishes while some people also prefer to have garlic turi with lukewarm water.

- **Ginger**

It is the ingredient which I love to add in my teas, be it black tea, green tea or milk tea due to its medicinal properties.

Key nutrients: Gingerol

Health benefits: natural remedy for nausea; helps with bloating and digestion, boosts the immune system and helps with cold and flu, it's anti-inflammatory and has anti-oxidant properties.

Ways to add ginger in your diet

- ✓ Drink ginger tea a few times a day.
- ✓ Add raw ginger to your smoothies

- **Kale or Leaf Cabbage**

This is one of miracle green leaf veggies which you must have been avoiding for years like me but trust me, after reading its health benefits, you will give it a chance.

Key nutrients: Vitamin C, sulforaphane, lutein, zeaxanthin antioxidant compounds, flavonoids like kaempferol and quercetin.

Health benefits: helps fight cancer, boosts eye health; helps fight free radicals, anti-viral, anti-inflammatory.

Ways to add it in your diet

- ✓ Use in salads or use it when cooking chicken, eggs or mix it with veggies.

- **Kidney beans**

This super food is almost everyone's favorite and one of the most delicious north Indian food delicacies.

Key nutrients: fiber, quality proteins for vegans and vegetarians, folate, iron, manganese, copper, and phosphorous

Health benefits of kidney beans: controls blood sugar, lowers cholesterol and reduces the risk of heart diseases. And yes, this super food has fantastic weight loss properties.

Ways to add it in your diet

- ✓ Make kidney beans in curry form or have boiled kidney beans salad.

- **Lentils**

So yes, let me admit this thing that lentils are a must for me every day as it is the best protein source and also it prolongs the period of hunger.

Key nutrients: fiber, folate, magnesium

Health benefits: lowers the risk of heart diseases, regulates blood circulation, slows the rate of digestion, stabilizes blood sugar, prevents neural tube defects in unborn babies due to folate, and aids in weight loss.

Ways to add it in your diet

- ✓ You can have cooked lentils, or knead the boiled lentils in flour and have lentil stuffed chapatti

- **Mung-bean sprouts**

This super food is very high in protein and fiber, so I always make sure that it is present in my salads every day.

Key nutrients: Potassium, Magnesium, Copper, Folate, Zinc

Health benefits: lowers inflammation, lower the risk of heart diseases, reduce the risk of cancer, and lowers the risk of diabetes.

Ways to add it in your diet

- ✓ Eat them as salads, or you can just have them roasted.

- **Chia Seeds**

My morning usually starts with this, as it has a high amount of antioxidants and a very high quality of protein in it.

Key nutrients: Calcium, Manganese, Magnesium, Phosphorous, Omega-3, Fiber

Health benefits: Chia seeds aid in weight loss due to fiber, loaded with antioxidants, and is good for bone health.

Ways to add it in your diet

- ✓ You can just blend them in your smoothies or have them soaked in the morning, or ground it and sprinkle over oatmeal or anything.

- **Buttermilk/ kefir/lassi**

It has the highest probiotic content in the world. Probiotics help in inhibiting the growth of various harmful bacteria.

Key nutrients: Calcium, Probiotics, Vitamin K2

Health benefits: inhibits the growth of various harmful bacteria like salmonella and E.coli, excellent for people suffering from IBS, and is good for bone health.

Ways to add it in your diet

- ✓ You can blend it with mint leaves and have this as summer coolers

So these all are some of the super foods which have immense benefits on your health. And also, if you incorporate these in your diet, they can do wonders for you. Just a few ingredients can help you complete your daily nutritional requirements and help your body to remain fit and healthy.

In the next and the last chapter, we will take a look at some questions we generally have in our mind while planning a diet.

PART IV - Questions and Answers

Chapter Twelve - Questions and Answers

Question 1: I usually catch a cold and have frequent infections. I doubt that I have a weak immune system. How can I boost my immune system? Which foods will help?

Answer: If you frequently catch cold, other various infections or you suffer from tummy problems like diarrhea etc. usually; there may be the signs of your weak immune system. To boost your immune system, you should include more of citrus fruits in your diet like oranges, grapefruit, lemons etc.

Vitamin C helps in boosting your immune system. You can also include vegetables like broccoli, spinach, ginger, garlic, bell peppers. Some seeds like sunflower seeds and nuts like almonds are rich in vitamin E, which is very important for regulating and maintaining immune system function. For a clearer picture of your problem, it is always advisable to consult a doctor.

Question 2: I have heard carbs make you fat. So for a week, I didn't have any carbs, but I feel weak and low on energy. Do all carbs make you fat?

Answer: If you are giving up all the carbs, you will lose weight but only for a temporary period. Later on, the weight you lost by giving up on carbs will more often return as fat. Not all the carbs are bad for you; you need to avoid only refined carbs if you want to lose weight faster. You will gain weight if you are consuming too many calories no matter whether they are coming from carbs, proteins or fats.

The adequate amount and right choice of every macronutrient are essential if you want healthy weight loss, otherwise you will look weak or sick. There are some good carbs which you can include in your weight loss diet; they are quinoa, lentils, beans, chickpeas, sweet potatoes, whole-grain cereals, oatmeal, barley, whole wheat bread, bananas, cherries, buckwheat etc.

Question 3: I am 25 years old and have a PCOS problem. I am 10kgs overweight. I have heard losing some weight can do wonders for PCOS. Can you tell me the foods that I need to involve or avoid in order to lose weight?

Answer: Every 1 in 10 women suffers from PCOS, i.e. polycystic ovary syndrome. It is a hormonal imbalance and metabolism problem that affects your overall health and appearance. Some women have lean PCOS, while others have obese PCOS. You have heard right losing weight can help in restoring the normal functions of ovaries and results in normal hormone production and result in improvement in symptoms also.

First of all, an exercise in any forms; be it walking, or yoga is essential for you and you should never give up on that. I recommend to avoid sugar strictly in any form just try to get sugar from fruits like apples, oranges etc. try to eat natural, fresh and local rather than processed. Avoid dairy and foods that have a high Glycemic index like pasta, white rice, bread, white potatoes, pastries, baked food. Cereals, etc., include gluten-free foods in your diet.

You can opt for:

- Coconut yoghurt, cruciferous vegetables, bitter greens, eggs, fatty fish including salmon, tuna etc., spinach, dried beans and lentils.
- Healthy fats like olive oil, coconut oil or avocado oil.

- Nuts like pistachios, walnuts, almonds, pine nuts.
- Spices like turmeric and cinnamon.

It is always to follow these foods after consulting your doctor.

Question 4: My gym instructor says there are 20mins window which gets open after your workout. Is it true? What foods do I need to eat before and after the training that will help me to gain muscle?

Answer: The window of opportunity as some people call it, will get opened immediately after your post-workout. It is said that your muscles are susceptible to accept the nutrients that help with strength; it is advisable to have your post-workout nutrition immediately and at most within 2 hours.

The more we delay in taking post-workout food, the more it will decrease the chances of muscle glycogen synthesis and protein storage when it comes to what to eat pre and post-workout. Then best foods to eat before your workout are you can have a protein bar, dried fruits and nuts, fruit and yoghurt, granola, a banana, whole-grain toast, oatmeal or a tablespoon of peanut butter.

Best foods to eat after your workout should involve protein to aid in protein synthesis and carbs to help in replacing muscle glycogen example: lean protein, eggs, vegetables, [protein shake or bar, avocado, hummus, fruit and yoghurt.

Question 5: I have heard that detoxification helps you in losing weight. Is it true? If yes, then how often should I detox?

Answer: Detoxification means eating lots of veggies, fruits and plenty of water. Detoxification may help you in losing weight. You will lose weight, but for a temporary period, all the weight loss will again come back as fat. People follow detox diets blindly, but it is similar to the other fad diets. Detoxification surely helps in the removal of harmful toxins that get accumulated in our body and which do not leave our body through urination and precipitation. Removal of toxins is essential to stay healthy and disease-free.

However, I would not recommend going on a detox diet as chances are of losing muscle mass, and you will gain lost weight once the diet is over. When it comes to how often you should detox, then it is a common practice to do a couple of detoxes a year, or whenever your skin is not doing good, or you have stomach issues, or you lack energy, or you have been eating a lot of processed foods since a while, then you should cleanse. Again I would say it depends on your lifestyle, and your current health, so doctor's advice is a must.

Question 6: I have a fatty liver, will boosting up metabolism help in curing fatty liver?

Answer: A healthy liver requires an adequate supply of both glycogen and triglycerides because, in retrieving the energy from triglycerides, the liver needs to burn some glycogen. What happens is the liver can easily make triglycerides as compared to glycogen. So when we continuously eat a high-fuel diet, the liver can clog up with triglycerides, leaving no room for glycogen.

Since the liver needs glycogen to burn triglycerides, the liver loses the ability to clear itself of the backlog of triglyceride fat. This results in what's called a fatty liver syndrome. It means that the liver is so overloaded with fat, that when new fuel comes in for processing, the liver is forced to send it away to be stored as body fat. In other words, we can say that a person who has fatty liver has a slow metabolism.

So definitely boosting your metabolism will do wonders. Some foods you can include in your diet as they have liver-aiding nutrients include: garlic, onions, radishes, fish, papaya, turmeric, tomatoes, grapes, and soy. All are packed with nutrients that help the liver break down its stores of fat.

Question 7: If I opt to follow a diet to lose weight, then for how long do I need to follow it?

Answer: Diet is a thing that aims at changing your lifestyle rather than only losing weight. So it is always advisable to choose a diet that suits your health status and also will provide you with the nutrients that your body will need. You may lose weight in 2 months or three months of following a diet, but the journey doesn't end here, after that, your diet will change to maintain the weight.

Diets do not only help you lose weight but helps to plan your cheat days effectively so that after losing your weight, you don't gain it back. What you can do is after following a diet for 2-3 months, you will get the idea about what to eat and how to eat, and you can then plan your schedule yourself without any extra help.

Question 8: If I don't include rice in my meals, will it help me in losing weight?

Answer: I don't recommend cutting down rice as it is part of a balanced diet. What matters is the number of calories. If you exceed your daily calorie intake, then that may add up to gaining weight. You should consume fewer calories than you burn to lose weight. Although calories in rice add up fast like 1 cup of cooked rice has 300 calories, but omitting rice is not the only way to cut your calories.

Here is one hack; don't take rice and roti together, because both grains have a high glycemic index and a very high carbohydrate intake. If you take them together, it leads to absorption of starch in your body leading to bloating and indigestion.

Question 9: Why should we eat every 2-3 hours if not hungry, won't it result in weight gain? How about skipping lunch if I had heavy breakfast?

Answer: Waiting to eat until you are hungry makes you eat more than required. Rather, eating wholesome, balanced meals or snacks every 2-3 hours will help will result in high metabolism which also leads to fat loss, helps you in stabilizing your blood sugar levels, and keep your energy levels high. So it is always advisable to distribute your daily calorie intake in 5-6 meals the entire day.

Try to include food from all groups like protein, fats, dairy, fruits, vegetables etc. since the lifestyle has become sedentary these days, like sitting on the office desk for hours. Hence, it is not advisable to have a heavy breakfast. And also it doesn't mean skipping your meals if you have eaten a lot in the morning. The best is to eat every 2-3 hours as large gaps between the meals can result in hyperacidity.

Question 10: I have a high cholesterol problem; can you tell me some good sources of fiber that will help me reduce my cholesterol levels?

Answer: Soluble fiber helps much in the absorption of cholesterol into your bloodstream. It is recommended that 5-10gms of serving of soluble fiber a day helps in decreasing your LDL cholesterol. Some easy ways to add extra fiber to your diet or meal plan are as follows:

- Before going to bed, you can have one tbsp of psyllium husk in one warm glass water.
- Flaxseeds are highly beneficial and are a great source of fiber, so you add them to your salad bowl, fruit bowl or in your dosa batter.
- Oat meals contain soluble fiber and a great breakfast option after your workout.
- Cereals like whole wheat bran flakes in milk can give you a sufficient amount of fiber.
- Apart from this, intake of salads, kidney beans, sprouts, fruits like apples and pears, avocados etc. are excellent sources of soluble fiber.

However, it is always advisable to consult your doctor before following any of these.

About the Author

I am an engineering graduate, a trained Kathak dancer, model, winner of MRS. DELHI NCR 2018, and a nutritionist. My journey as a nutritionist took the most crucial turn when I became a mother in 2019; I gained almost 20Kgs and weighed around 74Kgs.

I was depressed because I started feeling that my carrier in modeling was now a history. I tried everything from walking, running, and going to gym but with a baby, it was next to impossible. Finally, I took a call to plan my meals, keeping in mind the nutritional requirements of my baby and me as I was lactating.

This planned diet turned out to be game-changer for me and in a few months, I reduced 20 Kgs and came back to my pre-pregnancy weight, and that was when I started getting projects for various modeling assignments.

As quoted by Audrey Hepburn, *"As you grow older, you will discover that you have two hands- one for helping yourself, the other for helping others"*. From my own experience and helping several people in achieving a fit and healthy body, I decided to write a book which is, in general, can benefit all the people who are aiming to get back in shape or aiming for a healthy lifestyle on their own.

This book will help you in achieving your dream body, gaining confidence, fit in college jeans, look much younger than your age and stay fit without any gym, exercises or lifting heavyweights.

So stop waiting and worrying about those bulges and those extra Kgs; hold this book in your hands, understand your body and start being your diet planner and thus get back in your dream body.

Here I am, presenting this book to you all as I hope you read it, understand it and get back in better shape. You are most welcome to share your valuable feedback at:

thefitnesskey.diet@gmail.com

9 798559 273402